# 200 Low-Carb
# Slow Cooker Recipes

# 200 Low-Carb
# Slow Cooker Recipes

Healthy Dinners That Are Ready When You Are!

## Dana Carpender

FAIR WINDS
PRESS
GLOUCESTER, MASSACHUSETTS

First published in the USA in 2005 by
Fair Winds Press
33 Commercial Street
Gloucester, MA 01930

08 07 06 05 04  1 2 3 4 5

ISBN 1-59233-076-2

Library of Congress Cataloging-in-Publication Data available

Cover design by Mary Ann Smith
Book design by Leslie Haimes

Printed and bound in Canada

For my sister Kim,

who works way too hard,

and loves her slow cooker.

# CONTENTS

# Introduction:
# My Journey to Slow Cooker Mastery

I have a confession: When my editor, Holly, suggested I write a low-carb slow cooker book, I balked. Oh, I knew it would be popular—many readers had written me asking for a slow cooker book. I just wasn't thrilled at the idea of a couple of months of slow cooked dinners. I'd made some slow cooked meals that were pretty good, but overall, it seemed to me that most slow cooked food was not brilliant. Too many dishes seemed to be waterlogged, mushy, and insipid. Furthermore, so many slow cooker recipes seemed to rely on high-carb canned cream soups—indeed, many slow cooker books seemed to think that "put food in pot, dump in condensed cream of mushroom soup, and cook on low until you come home from work" was a recipe—but not in my book, figuratively or literally!

So I resisted for quite a while, but those e-mails saying, "Please, please, write us a slow cooker book!" were piling up in my inbox. I needed to write a slow cooker book! But it was clear I had to get better at slow cooking.

Well, my mom is a retired librarian, and I learned years ago that if you want to learn something, you need to look it up. So I went to Amazon.com and read reviews of slow cooker books to determine which were drawing raves. I then read the books that got the best reviews, gleaning what I could from them of the tricks of making slow cooker food as appealing as possible, both in taste and texture. Not surprisingly, my slow cooker performance took a remarkable upturn!

I also got an idea of what slow cookers do well. Obviously, they're not for anything that you want to come out crispy and brown, but if what you need is slow, moist cooking, a slow cooker will do it better than any other appliance. Preparing soups and stews and braising are obvious slow cooker strengths, but I also learned that a slow cooker is terrific for cooking anything that needs to be baked in a water bath (sometimes called a bain-marie)—custards, in particular. I was thrilled to discover that my slow cooker did the best job ever of roasting nuts and seeds, and it's perfect for hot beverages for parties and hors d'oeuvres that would otherwise need a chafing dish.

I was very surprised to learn that cooking fish in my slow cooker worked well. You can't leave it for hours and hours because fish overcooks easily. But just an hour or so of the gentle heat of the slow cooker leaves fish tender, moist, and succulent. Do try it when you have an hour to get dinner on the table, even if you mostly use your slow cooker to cook supper while you're out of the house for hours.

I also had a few spectacular failures. (Don't even ask about the brussels sprouts!) But overall, I was pleased to discover that with a few simple considerations in mind, slow cookers can turn out truly wonderful food.

## About Slow Cookers

By the time I finished this project, I owned three slow cookers. All of them are Rival Crock-Pots, the original slow cooker. (Crock-Pot is a brand name. All Crock-Pots are slow cookers, but not all slow cookers are Crock-Pots.) The Crock-Pot, as the original, is pretty much the gold standard of slow cookers. The heat comes from all around the crockery insert, rather than only coming from the bottom. If you have one of the slow cookers that has the heating element only on the bottom, you'll have to experiment a bit with these recipes to see if the times are correct.

The "low" setting on a Rival Crock-Pot is around 200°F (just above, actually, because things will boil eventually at this setting, and the boiling point is 212°F), and the "high" setting is around 300°F. If you have another brand of slow cooker that lets you set specific temperatures, keep this in mind. If you have another brand of slow cooker and you're not sure what temperature the settings will give (look in the booklet that came with it for this information), you can fill the slow cooker with water, heat it for 2 hours on low, and test the water's temperature with a kitchen thermometer, but this is a lot of trouble. I'd probably just use the low and high settings and keep mental notes on how meals turn out.

A good thing about the original Crock-Pot is that the crockery insert lifts out of the base. This allows it to be refrigerated, microwaved (if your microwave is big enough), and—most important—put in the dishwasher. *Do not* put your slow cooker in the dishwasher if the crockery cannot be separated from the heating element! Nothing electric should ever be submerged in water.

My slow cookers range in size. The smallest holds 2 1/2 quarts (2.5 liters), the middle-sized holds 3 quarts (3 liters), while the big one holds 5 1/2 quarts (5 liters). The 5 1/2-quart can easily hold enough food for 8 people. It's the obvious choice if you have a big family or like to cook enough to have leftovers for future meals. The 3-quart is the most common size. If you have a family of 4, it should be about right. If you have this size, figure you'll need to halve recipes that make 6 to 8 servings. The 2 1/2-quart is great for making dips, hot hors d'oeuvres, and hot beverages, but it is a bit small for family cooking.

Another consideration: My 5 1/2-quart Crock-Pot will fit a 6-cup casserole dish or 8" springform pan, opening up many new cooking options. If you have a smaller unit and want to make custards, cheesecakes, and other dishes that call for inserting a dish or pan, you'll have to find dishes that will fit. It's easier with a bigger slow cooker.

Keep in mind that slow cookers come in round or oval shapes. You'll want a round slow cooker, instead of an oval, so you can insert a round glass casserole or a springform. Sadly, a big, round slow cooker takes the most storage space. I know of no good way around this.

## Some Things I've Learned about Slow Cooking

- Browning meat or poultry before putting it in the slow cooker upgrades vast hordes of recipes. Yes, it takes time and dirties up a skillet. But the flavor and texture that browning bring are worth it, worth it, worth it. Often I'll have you sauté your vegetables, too.

- It's important to keep liquids to the minimum that will make the recipe work, especially in recipes that have a lot of vegetables. All of the liquid that cooks out of the food while slow cooking will accumulate in the pot because no evaporation occurs. It's easy to end up with very watery food. This rule does not apply to soups, of course.

- Because of this accumulation of liquid, it's a good idea to use concentrated flavors. In particular, you'll find that in many of these recipes I use both broth and bouillon concentrate to make what amounts to a broth that is double-strength or more.

- Sometimes it's a good idea to transfer the liquid from the slow cooker to a saucepan and boil it hard till it's reduced by half. Half the volume means double the flavor.

- It's generally best to use lean cuts of meat, and you'll see I've often used skinless poultry, too. This is because fat that becomes crackling and succulent in the oven makes slow cooker food unbearably greasy. This makes slow cooking a great way to cook some of the leaner and tougher cuts of meat that you might not want to roast. It also makes slow cooking a good cooking method for those of you who are watching calories as well as carbs. It can even save you money—often tough and bony cuts of meat are cheap.

- For some strange reason, vegetables cook more slowly in a slow cooker than meat does. If you put vegetables on top of the meat in your slow cooker, you may find that they're still crunchy when the rest of the dinner is done. Put the ingredients in the pot in the order given in the recipes in this book.

- For this reason, too, it's best to cut vegetables into fairly small pieces. You'll find I've told you what size to cut things, for the most part. If the recipe says 1/2" cubes, and you cut your turnips in 1 1/2" cubes, you're going to have underdone turnips.

- It's never a bad idea to spray your slow cooker with nonstick cooking spray before putting the food in it. I don't always do this, though I've specified it where it seems a particularly good idea. But I can't think of a situation in which it would hurt.

# Things That Other Slow Cooker Books Seem to Think Are Terribly Important, But Don't Seem Like a Big Deal to Me

- Several books wanted me to use only whole spices, such as whole peppercorns or coarse-cracked pepper, whole cloves, whole leaf herbs, etc., etc. I used what I had on hand. I got tasty food.

- A few books felt that you shouldn't season your slow cooker food until the end of cooking time. I do often suggest that you add salt and pepper to taste at the end of the cooking time, but other than that, our seasonings go into the pot with the food. I've never had a problem with this.

- Some books were emphatic about the size of the slow cooker. This matters some; you can't put 4 quarts of soup in a 3-quart slow cooker, and if you're only making a small batch of dip, you probably shouldn't use a 5 1/2-quart pot. But some cookbooks predicted dire results if I didn't fill my slow cooker at least halfway. I often filled my big slow cooker less than halfway. I got tasty food.

## About Timing

The biggest reason for the popularity of slow cookers is what I call "time-shifting"—the fact that they allow you to cook dinner at some time other than right before you eat it, so you can eat soon after you get home from work. Because of this, many slow cooker books tell you to cook most of their recipes for 8 hours or more. They figure you'll be away that long.

Unfortunately, I find that many dishes get unbearably mushy and overdone if they cook that long. I've tried to give the cooking times that I feel give the best results, which may not be the time that fits with your workday. These can generally be extended by an hour without a problem, but extending them by 2, 3, or more hours may well give you a very different result than I got.

A better idea is to do all your prep work the night before—cooking dinner after dinner, as it were. Then lift the filled crockery insert out of the base and stash it in the fridge overnight. The next morning, pull it out of the fridge, put it in the base, and turn it on, just before you leave the house. Starting with chilled food will add 1 to 2 hours to your cooking time. If you do this, don't heat up the base before putting the chilled crockery insert in! You may well crack the crockery.

If you need to extend your time even further, consider getting a timer. You should be fine letting your food wait 2 hours before the timer turns on the slow cooker—3 if the food is straight out of the fridge when the crockery goes in the base. It's a better idea to delay the starting time than to turn the pot off early because retained heat will cause the food to continue cooking even after the pot is turned off. Ask the nice people at your local hardware store about a timer you can plug things into. If you're just now acquiring your slow cooker, there are units available with time-delayed starters built in.

On the other hand, if you want to speed up a slow cooker recipe, you can do so by getting the contents warm before putting the crockery insert in the base. The crocks for two of my three slow cookers fit in my microwave. I have, on occasion, microwaved the crock on medium heat until it was warm through before putting the crock in the base to continue cooking. This cuts a good hour off the cooking time.

You can, of course, also use the high setting when the low setting is specified. This will cut the cooking time roughly in half. However, I find that for most recipes low yields better results. If you have the time to use it when it's recommended, I suggest you do so.

If you're going to be around for a while and leave the house later, you could cook on high for an hour or so, then switch to low when you leave. Figure, again, that each hour on high is worth 2 hours on low.

The size of your slow cooker relative to your recipe will somewhat affect the cooking time. If you have a 5 1/2-quart slow cooker and the food only fills it ¼ full, you can likely subtract 1 hour from the cooking time. Conversely, if the food fills your slow cooker to within an inch of the rim, you can add an hour.

# Ingredients
## Common and Not So Common Ingredients

Here, in alphabetical order, are a few ingredients I thought needed a little explanation:

- *Beer*—One or two recipes in this book call for beer. The lowest carbohydrate beer on the market is Michelob Ultra, but I don't much like it. Still, it should be okay for cooking. Miller Lite and Milwaukee's Best Light are better, and they have only about 0.5 grams more carb per can.

- *Black soybeans*—Most beans and other legumes are too high in carbohydrates for many low-carb dieters, but there is one exception. Black soybeans have a very low usable carb count, about 1 gram per serving, because most of the carbs in them are fiber. Several recipes in this book call for Eden brand canned black soybeans. Many health food stores carry these. If yours doesn't, I'll bet they could special order them for you. Health food stores tend to be wonderful about special orders.

  I wouldn't recommend eating soybean recipes several times a week. I know that soy has a reputation for being the Wonder Health Food of All Existence, but there are reasons to be cautious. For decades now, soy has been known to be hard on the thyroid, and if you're trying to lose weight and improve your health, a slow thyroid is the last thing you need. More alarmingly, a study done in Hawaii in 2000 showed a correlation between the amount of tofu subjects ate in middle age and their rate and severity of cognitive problems in old age. Because scientists suspect the problem lies with the soy estrogens that have been so highly touted, any unfermented soy product, including canned soybeans, is suspect.

  This doesn't mean we should completely shun soybeans and soy products, but we need to approach them with caution and eat them in moderation. Because many low-carb specialty products are soy-heavy, you'll want to pay attention there, too. Personally, I try to keep my soy consumption to 1 serving a week or less.

- **Blackstrap molasses**—What the heck is molasses doing in a low-carb cookbook?! It's practically all carbohydrate, after all. Well, yes, but I've found that combining Splenda with a very small amount of molasses gives a good, brown-sugar flavor to all sorts of recipes. Always use the darkest molasses you can find. The darker it is, the stronger the flavor, and the lower the carb count. That's why I specify blackstrap, the darkest, strongest molasses there is. It's nice to know that blackstrap is also where all the minerals they take out of sugar end up. It may be high-carb, but at least it's not a nutritional wasteland. Still, I use only small amounts.

  Most health food stores carry blackstrap molasses, but if you can't get it, buy the darkest molasses you can find. Most grocery store brands come in both light and dark varieties.

  Why not use some of the artificial brown-sugar flavored sweeteners out there? Because I've tried them, and I haven't tasted one I would be willing to buy again.

- **Broths**—Canned or boxed chicken broth and beef broth are very handy items to keep around and certainly quicker than making your own. However, the quality of most of the canned broth you'll find at your local grocery store is appallingly bad. The chicken broth has all sorts of chemicals in it, and often sugar as well. The beef broth is worse. It frequently has no beef in it whatsoever. I refuse to use these products, and you should, too.

  However, there are a few canned or boxed broths on the market worth buying. Many grocery stores now carry a brand called Kitchen Basics, which contains no chemicals at all. It is packaged in quart-size boxes, much like soy milk. Kitchen Basics comes in both chicken and beef. Health food stores also have good quality canned and boxed broths. Both Shelton and Health Valley brands are widely distributed in the United States.

  Decent packaged broth will cost you a little more than the stuff that is made of salt and chemicals, but not a whole lot more. If you watch for sales, you can often get it as cheaply as the bad stuff, so stock up. When my health food store runs a sale on good broth for 89 cents a can, I buy piles of it!

  **ONE LAST NOTE:** You will also find canned vegetable broth, particularly at health food stores. This is tasty, but because it runs much higher in carbohydrates than chicken and beef broths, I'd avoid it.

- ***Bouillon or broth concentrates*** — Bouillon or broth concentrate comes in cubes, crystals, liquids, and pastes. It is generally full of salt and chemicals and doesn't taste notably like the animal it supposedly came from. It definitely does *not* make a suitable substitute for good quality broth if you're making a pot of soup. However, these products can be useful for adding a little kick of flavor here and there — more as seasonings than as soups. For this use, I keep them on hand. I now use a paste bouillon concentrate product called Better Than Bouillon that comes in both chicken and beef flavors. I find it preferable to the granules or cubes.

- ***Carb Countdown dairy beverage*** — A very useful addition to low-carb cuisine is this carbohydrate-reduced milk product, available in full-fat, 2 percent, and skim, not to mention an exceedingly yummy chocolate variety. To me, Carb Countdown tastes just like milk, and I've used it pretty extensively in these recipes.

    I checked with the manufacturer, and Carb Countdown is nationally distributed, so you should be able to find it near you. However, if you cannot, try substituting half-and-half or equal parts of heavy cream and water. For that matter, if you're on the South Beach Diet, low-fat milk is allowed. Feel free to use it in place of Carb Countdown wherever I've specified it.

- ***Cauliflower*** — You'll notice a certain reliance on cauliflower in this book, both in the form of "Fauxtatoes" (see recipe page 239) and in the form of Cauli-Rice (see recipe page 239). This is because many slow cooker recipes make wonderful gravy, and it's a shame not to have a side dish to help you eat it. (Indeed, traditional slow cooker recipes show a similar dependence on potatoes, rice, and noodles.)

    You can skip the cauliflower if you like. Or you can substitute low-carb pasta from time to time, though I haven't found a brand I really like yet.

    **BY THE WAY:** If cauliflower (or another suggested garnish or side dish) isn't mentioned in the ingredient list, it's merely suggested and it's not included in the nutritional analysis for the dish. If it is in the ingredient list, it has been included in the analysis.

- ***Chili garlic paste*** — This is a traditional Asian ingredient, consisting mostly, as the name strongly implies, of hot chiles and garlic. If, like me, you're a chile-head, you'll find endless ways to use the stuff once you have it on hand. Chili garlic paste comes in jars, and it keeps for months in the refrigerator. It is worth seeking out at Asian markets or in the international foods aisle of big grocery stores.

- *Chipotle peppers canned in adobo sauce*—Chipotle peppers are smoked jalapeños. They're very different from regular jalapeños, and they're quite delicious. Look for them, canned in adobo sauce, in the Mexican foods section of big grocery stores. Because you're unlikely to use the whole can at once, you'll be happy to know that you can store your chipotles in the freezer, where they'll keep for months. I just float my can in a bowl of hot tap water for 5 minutes till it's thawed enough to peel off one or two peppers, then put it right back in the freezer.

- *Fish sauce or nuoc mam or nam pla*—This is a salty, fermented seasoning widely used in Southeast Asian cooking, available in Asian grocery stores and in the Asian food sections of big grocery stores. Grab it when you find it; it keeps nicely without refrigeration. Fish sauce is used in a few (really great) recipes in this book, and it adds an authentic flavor. In a pinch, you can substitute soy sauce, although you'll lose some of the Southeast Asian accent.

- *Garlic*—I use only fresh garlic, except for occasional recipes for sprinkle-on seasoning blends. Nothing tastes like the real thing. To my taste buds, even the jarred, chopped garlic in oil doesn't taste like fresh garlic. We won't even *talk* about garlic powder. You may use jarred garlic if you like—half a teaspoon should equal about 1 clove of fresh garlic. If you choose to use powdered garlic, well, I can't stop you, but I'm afraid I can't promise the recipes will taste the same either. One quarter teaspoon of garlic powder is the rough equivalent of 1 clove of fresh garlic.

- *Ginger root*—Many recipes in this book call for fresh ginger, sometimes called ginger root. Dried, powdered ginger is *not* a substitute. Fortunately, fresh ginger freezes beautifully. Drop the whole ginger root (called a hand of ginger) into a resealable plastic freezer bag, and toss it in the freezer. When time comes to use it, pull it out, peel enough of the end for your immediate purposes, and grate it. Ginger grates just fine while still frozen. Throw the remaining root back in the bag and toss it back in the freezer.

  Ground fresh ginger root in oil is available in jars at some very comprehensive grocery stores. I buy this when I can find it without added sugar, but otherwise, I grate my own.

- *Guar and xanthan gums*—These sound just dreadful, don't they? But they're in lots of your favorite processed foods, so how bad can they be? They're forms of water soluble fiber, extracted and purified. Guar and xanthan are both flavorless white powders, and their value to us is as low-carb thickeners. Technically speaking, these are carbs, but they're all fiber. Nothing but.

Those of you who read *500 Low-Carb Recipes* know that I used to recommend putting your guar or xanthan through the blender with part or all of the liquid in the recipe, to avoid lumps. You may now happily forget that technique. Instead, acquire an extra salt shaker, fill it with guar or xanthan, and keep it handy. When you want to thicken the liquid in your slow cooker, simply sprinkle a little of the thickener over the surface *while stirring*, preferably with a whisk. Stop when your sauce, soup, or gravy is a little less thick than you want it to be. It'll thicken a little more on standing.

Your health food store may well be able to order guar or xanthan for you if they don't have them on hand. You can also find suppliers online. Of the two, I slightly prefer xanthan.

- **Ketatoes**—Ketatoes is a low-carb version of instant mashed potatoes. It actually contains some dehydrated potato, diluted with a lot of fiber. You simply mix the powder with equal amounts of water.

  Or not. Personally, I find Ketatoes made according to the package directions unappealing. They smell good, but the texture is off. However, used in small quantities, Ketatoes mix allows us to give a convincingly potato flavor to a variety of dishes. I've used Ketatoes mix in a number of the recipes in this book. Be aware that Ketatoes come in a variety of flavors, but all my recipes call for Ketatoes Classic—plain potato flavor.

  If you can't buy Ketatoes in your hometown, there are about a billion online merchants who would be happy to ship them to you.

- **Low-carb tortillas**—These are becoming easier and easier to find. I can get them at every grocery store in town. If you can't buy them at a local store, you can order them online. They keep pretty well. I've had them hang around for 3 or 4 weeks in a sealed bag without getting moldy or stale, so you might want to order more than one package at a time.

  I use La Tortilla Factory brand because they've got the lowest usable carb count of any I've found, just 3 grams. They're mostly made of fiber! Beware: I have recently seen "low-carb" tortillas with deceptive packaging. The listed serving size turned out to equal only half of one tortilla. That's not a serving, as far as I'm concerned!

- **Low-sugar preserves**—In particular, I find low-sugar apricot preserves to be a wonderfully versatile ingredient. I buy Smucker's brand and like it very much. This is lower in sugar by *far* than the "all fruit" preserves, which replace sugar with concentrated fruit juice. Folks, sugar from fruit juice is still sugar. I also have been known to use low-sugar orange marmalade and low-sugar raspberry preserves.

- **Splenda**—Be aware that Splenda granular that comes in bulk, in a box, or in the new "baker's bag" is different than the Splenda that comes in the little packets. The Splenda in the packets is considerably sweeter. One packet equals 2 teaspoons granular Splenda. All these recipes use granular Splenda.

- **Sugar-free imitation honey**—This is a polyol (sugar alcohol) syrup with flavoring added to make it taste like honey. The two brands I've tried, one by HoneyTree and the other by Steele's, are not bad imitations.

  Sugar-free imitation honey is becoming more and more available, and it is a useful product. I can get sugar-free imitation honey here in Bloomington at Sahara Mart, my favorite source of low-carb specialty products, and I've heard from readers that Wal-Mart now carries it. For that matter, many of the low-carb e-tailers carry Steele's brand of imitation honey. It shouldn't be too hard to get your hands on some.

- **Sugar-free pancake syrup**—This is actually easy to find. All my local grocery stores carry it—indeed, many have more than one brand. It's usually with the regular pancake syrup, but it may be shelved with the diabetic or diet foods. It's just like regular pancake syrup, only it's made from polyols (sugar alcohols) instead of sugar. I use it in small quantities in a few recipes to get a maple flavor.

- **Vege-Sal**—If you've read my newsletter, *Lowcarbezine!* or my previous cookbooks, you know that I'm a big fan of Vege-Sal. It's a salt that's been seasoned, but don't think "seasoned salt." Vege-Sal is much milder than traditional seasoned salt. It's simply salt that's been blended with some dried, powdered vegetables. The flavor is quite subtle, but I think it improves all sorts of things. I've given you the choice between using regular salt or Vege-Sal in many recipes. Don't worry, they'll come out fine with plain old salt, but I do think Vege-Sal adds a little something extra. Vege-Sal is made by Modern Products, and it is widely available in health food stores.

# CHAPTER ONE

# Slow Cooker Snacks and Hot Hors D'oeuvres

Slow cookers are mostly used for cooking dinner while you're out of the house, but they have other uses, such as keeping hors d'oeuvres and dips hot through your whole party! Plus your slow cooker will do the best job of roasting nuts ever. Here are some ways you can make your slow cooker the life of the party.

##  Glazed Chicken Wings

Put out a pot of these and a big ol' pile of napkins and watch your guests eat!

> 3 pounds (1.5 kilograms) chicken wings
> 1/2 cup (170 grams) sugar-free imitation honey
> 1/2 cup (12 grams) Splenda
> 1/2 cup (120 milliliters) soy sauce
> 2 tablespoons (28 milliliters) oil
> 2 cloves garlic
> 2 tablespoons (15 grams) Dana's No-Sugar Ketchup (see recipe page 228)
>    or purchased low-carb ketchup

Cut the chicken wings into "drummettes." Season them with salt and pepper and put them in your slow cooker.

In a bowl, stir together the honey, Splenda, soy sauce, oil, garlic, and ketchup. Drizzle the mixture over the wings and stir them to coat. Cover the slow cooker, set it to low, and let it cook for 6 to 8 hours.

**YIELD:** 8 servings, each with: 144 calories, 10 g fat, 10 g protein, 2 g carbohydrate, trace dietary fiber, 2 g usable carbs. (Counts do not include the polyols in the imitation honey.)

#  Cranberry-Barbecue Meatballs

Boring old ground turkey does a Cinderella turn and comes to the party in this dish!

2 pounds (1 kilogram) ground turkey

2 eggs

4 scallions, minced

2 tablespoons (28 milliliters) soy sauce

1/4 teaspoon orange extract

1/2 teaspoon pepper

1 teaspoon Splenda

1/4 cup (60 milliliters) oil

1 cup (235 milliliters) low-carb barbecue sauce (see recipe page 231 or purchase)

1 cup (110 grams) cranberries (These are strictly seasonal, but they freeze well.)

1/4 cup (6 grams) Splenda

In a big mixing bowl, combine the turkey, eggs, and scallions.

In another bowl, mix together the soy sauce, orange extract, pepper, and 1 teaspoon Splenda and pour into the bowl with the turkey. Now use clean hands to smoosh it all together until it's very well blended. Make 1" (25 millimeter) meatballs from the mixture.

Heat half the oil in a big, heavy skillet over medium heat. Brown the meatballs in a few batches, adding the rest of the oil as needed. Transfer the browned meatballs to your slow cooker.

In a blender or food processor with an S-blade, combine the barbecue sauce, cranberries, and 1/4 cup Splenda. Run it until the berries are pureed. Pour this mixture over the meatballs. Cover the slow cooker, set to low, and let it cook for 5 to 6 hours. Serve hot from the slow cooker with toothpicks for spearing!

YIELD: 48 meatballs, each with: 44 calories, 3 g fat, 4 g protein, 1 g carbohydrate, trace dietary fiber, 1 g usable carbs.

# Colombo Meatballs with Jerk Sauce

Colombo is the Caribbean version of curry, and jerk is the notoriously fiery barbecue marinade from Jamaica. The heat of this recipe is best controlled by choosing your hot sauce wisely. Use Tabasco, or Louisiana hot sauce, and they'll be spicy. Use Jamaican Scotch Bonnet sauce, or habanero sauce, and they'll take the top of your head right off!

1 pound (455 grams) ground lamb

1 egg

1/4 cup (40 grams) minced onion

1/4 teaspoon ground coriander

1/4 teaspoon ground turmeric

1/8 teaspoon anise seed, ground

1 clove garlic, minced

1/4 teaspoon dry mustard

2 teaspoons lemon juice

1/2 teaspoon Splenda

1/2 teaspoon salt

2 tablespoons (28 milliliters) olive oil

1 bay leaf

1/4 cup (40 grams) minced onion

1 teaspoon ground allspice

1 tablespoon (8 grams) grated ginger root

1 tablespoon (14 milliliters) soy sauce

1/4 teaspoon dried thyme

1/4 teaspoon ground cinnamon

1 tablespoon (1.5 grams) Splenda

2 cloves garlic, crushed

1/4 cup (60 grams) low-carb ketchup

1 tablespoon (14 milliliters) lemon juice

1 tablespoon (14 milliliters) lime juice

1 1/2 teaspoons hot sauce

In a big mixing bowl, add the lamb, egg, 1/4 cup minced onion, coriander, turmeric, anise seed, minced garlic, dry mustard, 2 teaspoons lemon juice, 1/2 teaspoon Splenda, and salt. Using clean hands, moosh it all together till it's well blended. Then make 1" (25 millimeters) meatballs, pressing them together firmly.

Heat the oil in a big, heavy skillet over medium heat and brown the meatballs in two batches. Drop the bay leaf in the bottom of the slow cooker, then put the meatballs on top of it.

Mix together the second 1/4 cup minced onion, the allspice, ginger, soy sauce, thyme, cinnamon, 1 tablespoon Splenda, crushed garlic, ketchup, 1 tablespoon lemon juice, lime juice, and hot sauce. Pour this sauce evenly over the meatballs. Cover the slow cooker, set it to low, and let it cook for 3 hours. Serve hot from the slow cooker.

**YIELD:** 35 servings, each with: 48 calories, 4 g fat, 2 g protein, 1 g carbohydrate, trace dietary fiber, 1 g usable carbs.

# 🍲 Easy Party Shrimp

How easy is this?! Yet your guests will devour it. If you can't find the crab boil spices in the spice aisle at your grocery store, ask the fish guys. They should know where it is.

    1 envelope (3 ounces/85 grams) crab boil spices
    12 ounces (355 milliliters) light beer
    1 tablespoon (18 grams) salt or Vege-Sal
    4 pounds (2 kilograms) easy-peel shrimp or frozen shrimp, unthawed

Drop the crab boil spice net bag in your slow cooker and pour in the beer. Add the salt or Vege-Sal and stir. Add the shrimp. Add just enough water to bring the liquid level up to the top of the shrimp. Cover the slow cooker, set it to high, and let it cook for 1 to 2 hours, until the shrimp are pink through. Set the pot to low.

Serve the shrimp straight from the slow cooker with low-carb cocktail sauce, lemon butter, or mustard and mayo stirred together, for dipping. Or heck, all three. This is enough shrimp for a good-sized party, at least 15 or 20 people, if you're serving it as an hors d'oeuvre/party snack.

**YIELD:** 20 servings, each with: 101 calories, 2 g fat, 18 g protein, 1 g carbohydrate, 0 g dietary fiber, 1 g usable carbs. (Analysis does not include any dipping sauces.)

# Zippy Cocktail Dogs

Here's an easy way to jazz up little cocktail wieners.

    1/4 cup (60 grams) Dana's No-Sugar Ketchup (see recipe page 228)
        or purchased low-carb ketchup
    1/4 cup (6 grams) Splenda
    1/2 teaspoon blackstrap molasses
    1 teaspoon Worcestershire sauce
    1/4 cup (60 milliliters) bourbon
    1/2 pound (225 grams) cocktail-size hot dogs

In a large bowl, stir together the ketchup, Splenda, molasses, Worcestershire sauce, and bourbon.

Put the hot dogs in the slow cooker and pour the sauce over them. Cover the slow cooker, set it to low, and let it cook for 2 hours, then uncover and cook for 1 more hour. Serve with toothpicks for spearing.

**NOTE:** If you can't get cocktail-size hot dogs, use regular hot dogs cut in chunks. They're not as cute, but they should taste the same!

**YIELD:** 6 servings, each with: 158 calories, 11 g fat, 5 g protein, 4 g carbohydrate, trace dietary fiber, 4 g usable carbs.

# Horseradish Smokies

My husband loved these!

 1 pound (455 grams) small smoked sausage links

 $^1/4$ cup (60 grams) Dana's No-Sugar Ketchup (see recipe page 228)
  or purchased low-carb ketchup

 $^1/3$ cup (8 grams) Splenda

 2 tablespoons (30 grams) prepared horseradish

 $^1/4$ teaspoon blackstrap molasses

Put the sausage in your slow cooker.

In a bowl, mix the ketchup, Splenda, horseradish, and molasses. Pour the sauce over the sausage. Stir to coat the sausage. Cover the slow cooker, set it to low, and let it cook for 3 hours. Serve the sausage hot from the slow cooker with toothpicks for spearing.

**YIELD:** 8 servings, each with: 193 calories, 17 g fat, 8 g protein, 1 g carbohydrate, trace dietary fiber, 1 g usable carbs.


# Orange Smokies

Put these out at your next Super Bowl party and watch people eat!

 1 pound (455 grams) small smoked sausage links

 $^1/4$ cup (60 grams) Dana's No-Sugar Ketchup (see recipe page 228)
  or purchased low-carb ketchup

 $^1/4$ cup (60 milliliters) lemon juice

 2 tablespoons (3 grams) Splenda

 $^1/4$ teaspoon orange extract

 $^1/4$ teaspoon guar or xanthan (optional)

Put the sausage in your slow cooker.

In a small bowl, stir together the ketchup, lemon juice, Splenda, and orange extract. Thicken the mixture just a little, if you think it needs it, with guar or xanthan. Pour the sauce over the sausage. Cover the slow cooker, set it to low, and let it cook for 3 hours. Keep the sausages hot in the slow cooker to serve.

**YIELD:** 8 servings, each with: 193 calories, 17 g fat, 8 g protein, 1 g carbohydrate, trace dietary fiber, 1 g usable carbs.

# Bacon-Cheese Dip

Bacon and cheese together. Just makes you glad to be a low-carber, doesn't it?

16 ounces (455 grams) Neufchâtel cheese, softened, or light
  or regular cream cheese
2 cups (225 grams) shredded cheddar cheese
2 cups (230 grams) shredded Monterey Jack cheese
1/2 cup (120 milliliters) Carb Countdown dairy beverage
1/2 cup (120 milliliters) heavy cream
2 tablespoons (30 grams) brown mustard
1 tablespoon (10 grams) minced onion
2 teaspoons Worcestershire sauce
1/2 teaspoon salt or Vege-Sal
1/4 teaspoon cayenne
1 pound (455 grams) bacon, cooked, drained, and crumbled

Cut the Neufchâtel cheese or cream cheese in cubes and put them in your slow cooker. Add the cheddar cheese, Monterey Jack cheese, Carb Countdown, cream, mustard, onion, Worcestershire sauce, salt or Vege-Sal, and cayenne. Stir to distribute the ingredients evenly. Cover the slow cooker, set it to low, and let it cook for 1 hour, stirring from time to time.

When the cheese has melted, stir in the bacon.

**NOTE:** Serve with cut-up vegetables, fiber crackers, or other low-carb dippers.

**YIELD:** 12 servings, each with: 505 calories, 44 g fat, 25 g protein, 2 g carbohydrate, trace dietary fiber, 2 g usable carbs.

# Bagna Cauda

The name of this traditional Italian dip means "hot bath," and that's just what it is—a bath of hot, flavored olive oil to dip your vegetables in. Believe it or not, our tester Maria Vander Vloedt's kids really liked this!

1 cup (235 milliliters) extra-virgin olive oil

1/4 cup (55 grams) butter

3 cloves garlic, minced

2 ounces (55 grams) canned anchovies, minced

Combine everything in a small slow cooker. Cover the slow cooker, set it to low, and let it cook for 1 hour.

**NOTE:** Serve with vegetables. Fennel, pepper strips, cauliflower, mushrooms, celery, canned artichoke hearts, and lightly steamed asparagus are all traditional choices.

**YIELD:** Per batch: 2448 calories, 267 g fat, 17 g protein, 3 g carbohydrate, trace dietary fiber, 3 g usable carbs. (It's hard to know how to divide this into servings, and it's unlikely you'll end up eating it all, even with a big group. After all, you can't scoop up a tablespoon at a time of hot olive oil. So here's the stats for the whole potful. Notice that carb count!)

# Hot Artichoke Dip

This is my slow cooker version of the ubiquitous hot artichoke dip that appeared in *500 Low-Carb Recipes*. Using a slow cooker, the dip stays hot till it's gone!

    1 cup (225 grams) mayonnaise
    1 cup (100 grams) grated Parmesan cheese
    1 clove garlic, crushed
    8 ounces (225 grams) shredded mozzarella cheese
    14 ounces (400 grams) canned artichoke hearts, drained and chopped

Add everything to your slow cooker, stir it up well, and smooth the surface. Cover the slow cooker, set it to low, and let it cook for 2 to 3 hours.

Serve with low-carb crackers and/or cut-up vegetables.

**YIELD:** 8 servings, each with: 339 calories, 33 g fat, 11 g protein, 2 g carbohydrate, 1 g dietary fiber, 1 g usable carbs.

# Hot Crab Dip

Hot crab, hot cheese, garlic—what's not to like?

    1 cup (225 grams) mayonnaise
    8 ounces (225 grams) shredded cheddar cheese
    4 scallions, minced
    6 ounces (170 grams) canned crabmeat, drained
    1 clove garlic, crushed
    3 ounces (85 grams) cream cheese, softened, cut into chunks

Combine everything in your slow cooker and stir together. Cover the slow cooker, set it to low, and let it cook for 1 hour. Remove the lid and stir to blend in the now-melted cream cheese. Re-cover and cook for another hour.

Serve with celery, pepper, and cucumber dippers

**YIELD:** 8 servings, each with: 372 calories, 37 g fat, 13 g protein, 1 g carbohydrate, trace dietary fiber, 1 g usable carbs.

# ⌐•⌐ Artichoke-Spinach-Ranch Dip

Artichoke dip, spinach dip, and ranch dip are all so popular, combining them seemed destined for greatness!

14 ounces (400 grams) canned artichoke hearts, drained and chopped

10 ounce (280 gram) package frozen chopped spinach, thawed and drained

1 cup (225 grams) mayonnaise

1 cup (230 grams) sour cream

1 packet (1 ounce/28 grams) ranch-style dressing mix

2 cups (160 grams) shredded Parmesan cheese

1 clove garlic, crushed

Spray your slow cooker with nonstick spray. Mix everything together in your slow cooker. Cover, set it to low, and let it cook for 3 to 4 hours. Keep the dip hot in the slow cooker to serve.

**NOTE:** Serve dip with cut-up vegetables or low-carb crackers.

**YIELD:** 12 servings, each with: 247 calories, 23 g fat, 7 g protein, 4 g carbohydrate, 1 g dietary fiber, 3 g usable carbs.

# Chicken Liver Pâté

If you like chicken livers, you'll like this, but you won't if you don't. I adore them myself and practically lived on pâté on fiber crackers for a few days after making this. You could also stuff this into celery stalks.

1/2 cup (65 grams) finely chopped onion

1 clove garlic, crushed

1 cup (100 grams) sliced mushrooms

3 tablespoons (45 grams) butter

1 pound (455 grams) chicken livers

2 tablespoons (28 milliliters) heavy cream

2 tablespoons (28 milliliters) brandy

1 bay leaf, crumbled

1/2 teaspoon dried thyme

1/2 teaspoon dried marjoram

1 tablespoon (4 grams) chopped fresh parsley

3/4 teaspoon salt or Vege-Sal

1/2 teaspoon pepper

In a big, heavy skillet, start the onion, garlic, and mushrooms sautéing in the butter over low heat. While that's happening, halve the chicken livers where they naturally divide into two lobes. When the mushrooms have softened and changed color, add the livers and sauté, stirring occasionally, until they're sealed all over and the color of the surface has changed, but they are not cooked through. Transfer the mixture to a food processor with the S-blade in place.

Add the cream, brandy, bay leaf, thyme, marjoram, parsley, salt or Vege-Sal, and pepper. Run the food processor until the mixture is finely pureed.

Spray a 3- or 4-cup (710-945 ml) glass casserole dish with nonstick cooking spray. Pour the mixture from the food processor into the casserole dish. Place the casserole dish in your slow cooker. Carefully pour water around the casserole dish to within 1" of the rim. Cover the slow cooker, set it to low, and let it cook for 8 hours, or until the mixture is well set. Turn off the slow cooker and let the water cool until you can remove the casserole dish without risk of scalding your fingers. Remove the casserole dish and chill the pâté overnight before serving.

You can simply scoop this from the casserole dish with a knife and spread it on fiber crackers if you like, but it's fancier to turn it out, slice it, and serve it on a bed of greens.

**YIELD:** 8 servings, each with: 138 calories, 8 g fat, 11 g protein, 4 g carbohydrate, trace dietary fiber, 4 g usable carbs.

# Roasted Nuts and Seeds

I was astounded by how great a job my slow cooker did of roasting nuts! I got a little carried away, I confess. But then, I really like nuts! Make these often and keep them on hand, and you'll find yourself missing both chips and candy a whole lot less.

## ⊡ Dana's Snack Mix, Slow Cooker–Style

This is similar to a snack mix that appears in *500 Low-Carb Recipes*, and it's addictive. Thank goodness it's also healthy! You'll likely find shelled pumpkin seeds and raw, shelled sunflower seeds at your health food store. You can also find the pumpkin seeds in Latino groceries, labeled "pepitas."

> 4 tablespoons (55 grams) butter, melted
>
> 3 tablespoons (50 grams) Worcestershire sauce
>
> 1 1/2 teaspoons garlic powder
>
> 2 1/2 teaspoons seasoned salt
>
> 2 teaspoons onion powder
>
> 2 cups (450 grams) raw pumpkin seeds, shelled
>
> 1 cup (225 grams) raw sunflower seeds, shelled
>
> 1 cup (145 grams) raw almonds
>
> 1 cup (100 grams) raw pecans
>
> 1 cup (125 grams) raw walnut pieces
>
> 1 cup (130 grams) raw cashews
>
> 1 cup (145 grams) dry-roasted peanuts

If you've got a little time, you can just put the butter in the slow cooker, turn it to low, and wait for it to melt. Otherwise, melt it on the stove or in the microwave, and then transfer it to the slow cooker pot. Add the Worcestershire sauce, garlic powder, seasoned salt, and onion powder. Stir it all together. Add the nuts and seeds. Stir well, until all the nuts are evenly coated. Cover the slow cooker, set it to low, and let it cook for 5 to 6 hours, stirring once or twice if you're around.

Uncover the pot, stir the nut and seed mix up, and cook for another 45 to 60 minutes to dry the nuts and seeds. Let them cool before storing them in an airtight container.

**YIELD:** 24 servings of 1/3 cup, each with: 279 calories, 25 g fat, 9 g protein, 9 g carbohydrate, 3 g dietary fiber, 6 g usable carbs.

# Blue Cheese Dressing Walnuts

I originally wanted to make these with powdered blue cheese dressing mix, only to find that there is no such thing, at least not in my grocery stores. So I tried using liquid dressing instead. It didn't end up tasting a lot like blue cheese, but it did end up tasting really good.

4 cups (400 grams) walnuts
1/2 cup (120 milliliters) blue cheese salad dressing
1 teaspoon garlic salt

Combine the walnuts and dressing in your slow cooker. Stir until the nuts are evenly coated with the dressing. Cover the slow cooker, set it to low, and let it cook for 3 hours, stirring once halfway through.

Stir in the garlic salt just before serving.

**YIELD:** 16 servings, each with: 228 calories, 22 g fat, 8 g protein, 4 g carbohydrate, 2 g dietary fiber, 2 g usable carbs.

# Cajun-Spiced Pecans

You can used purchased Cajun seasoning for this or make your own from the recipe on page 235.

1 pound (455 grams) pecan halves
2 tablespoons (28 grams) butter, melted
3 tablespoons (18 grams) Cajun seasoning

Place the pecans in your slow cooker. Stir in the butter to coat the pecans. Add the Cajun seasoning and stir again to coat. Cover the slow cooker, set it to low, and let it cook for 3 hours, stirring once halfway through if you are around.

**YIELD:** 16 servings, each with: 118 calories, 12 g fat, 1 g protein, 4 g carbohydrate, 1 g dietary fiber, 3 g usable carbs.

# Candied Pecans

These are a great treat to leave around in pretty little dishes at a holiday party.

1 pound (100 grams) pecan halves

$^1/_2$ cup (112 grams) butter, melted

$^1/_2$ cup (12 grams) Splenda

1 $^1/_2$ teaspoons ground cinnamon

$^1/_4$ teaspoon ground ginger

$^1/_4$ teaspoon ground allspice

Put the pecans in your slow cooker and stir in the melted butter, coating the pecans thoroughly. Sprinkle the Splenda, cinnamon, ginger, and allspice over the pecans and stir again to coat.

Cover the slow cooker, set it to high, let it cook for 30 minutes. Then uncover, turn it to low, and let it cook for 1 $^1/_2$ to 2 hours.

**YIELD:** 8 servings, each with: 304 calories, 32 g fat, 2 g protein, 6 g carbohydrate, 3 g dietary fiber, 3 g usable carbs.

# Kickin' Pecans

This isn't enough cayenne to be really hot, just enough to add a little kick. Hence the name.

> 3 cups (300 grams) pecan halves
>
> 1 egg white
>
> 1 teaspoon cinnamon
>
> 1/2 teaspoon salt
>
> 1/4 teaspoon cayenne, or more to taste
>
> 1 cup (25 grams) Splenda

Put the pecans in your slow cooker. Add the egg white and stir until the pecans are evenly coated.

In a bowl, stir together the cinnamon, salt, cayenne, and Splenda. Pour the mixture over the pecans and stir until they're evenly coated. Cover the slow cooker, set it to low, and let it cook for 3 hours, stirring every hour or so.

If the nuts aren't dry by the end of the 3 hours, uncover the slow cooker, stir, and cook for another 30 minutes until dry. Store in an airtight container.

**YIELD:** 9 servings, each with: 242 calories, 24 g fat, 3 g protein, 7 g carbohydrate, 3 g dietary fiber, 4 g usable carbs.

# Curried Pecans

These are astonishingly good. I may make them in quantity and give them away for Christmas this year!

3 tablespoons (45 grams) butter

1/4 teaspoon blackstrap molasses

1 1/2 teaspoons curry powder

1/4 teaspoon salt

1/4 teaspoon ground cumin

12 ounces (340 grams) pecan halves

2 tablespoons (3 grams) Splenda

In a big, heavy skillet, melt the butter over medium-low heat. Stir in the molasses, curry powder, salt, and cumin and cook for just a minute or two.

Add the pecans and stir until they're evenly coated with the butter and seasonings. Then transfer them to your slow cooker. Sprinkle the Splenda over the pecans, stirring as you sprinkle, so you coat them evenly. Cover the slow cooker, set it to low, and let it cook for 2 to 3 hours, stirring once or twice during the cooking time.

YIELD: 9 servings, each with: 169 calories, 17 g fat, 2 g protein, 4 g carbohydrate, 2 g dietary fiber, 2 g usable carbs.

# Smokin' Chili Peanuts

Oh, my goodness. These are hot and crunchy and just too darned good. But they're not for the faint of heart.

> 1/4 cup (55 grams) butter, melted
> 2 tablespoons (15 grams) chili powder
> 1 tablespoon (14 milliliters) liquid smoke flavoring
> 24 ounce (680 gram) jar salted, dry-roasted peanuts

In your slow cooker, combine the butter, chili powder, and liquid smoke flavoring. Stir them together well. Add the peanuts and stir them until they're evenly coated with the butter and the seasonings. Cover the slow cooker, set it to low, and let it cook for 2 to 2 1/2 hours.

Remove the lid, stir, and let cook for another 30 minutes or until the peanuts are dry. Store 'em in the original jar!

**YIELD:** 24 servings, each with: 185 calories, 16 g fat, 7 g protein, 6 g carbohydrate, 2 g dietary fiber, 4 g usable carbs.

# Butter-Spice Almonds

> 3 cups (435 grams) almonds
> 2 tablespoons (28 grams) butter, melted
> 2 teaspoons vanilla extract
> 2 teaspoons butter-flavored extract
> 1/2 cup (12 grams) Splenda
> 1 teaspoon ground cinnamon
> 1/4 teaspoon salt

Put the almonds in your slow cooker.

In a bowl, stir together the butter, vanilla extract, and butter-flavored extract until well combined. Pour the mixture over the almonds and stir to coat. Add the Splenda, cinnamon, and salt and stir to coat again. Cover the slow cooker, set it to low, and let it cook for 4 to 5 hours, stirring once or twice.

When the time's up, uncover the slow cooker, stir the almonds again, and let them cook for another 30 to 45 minutes. Store in an airtight container.

**YIELD:** 6 servings, each with: 457 calories, 41 g fat, 14 g protein, 15 g carbohydrate, 8 g dietary fiber, 7 g usable carbs.

# Maple-Glazed Walnuts

3 cups (300 grams) walnuts

1 1/2 teaspoons ground cinnamon

1 tablespoon (14 grams) butter, melted

1/4 teaspoon salt

2 teaspoons vanilla extract

1/3 cup (78 milliliters) sugar-free pancake syrup

1/3 cup (8 grams) Splenda

Put the walnuts in your slow cooker.

In a bowl, mix together the cinnamon, butter, salt, vanilla extract, pancake syrup, and 1/4 cup of the Splenda. Pour the mixture over the nuts and stir to coat. Cover the slow cooker, set it to low, and let it cook for 2 to 3 hours, stirring every hour or so.

Then uncover the slow cooker and cook, stirring every 20 minutes, until the nuts are almost dry. Stir in the remaining 2 tablespoons Splenda, cook for another 20 minutes, then remove from the slow cooker and cool. Store in an airtight container.

**YIELD:** 9 servings, each with: 268 calories, 25 g fat, 10 g protein, 6 g carbohydrate, 2 g dietary fiber, 4 g usable carbs.

# CHAPTER TWO

# Slow Cooker Eggs

Eggs cook so quickly, it seems odd to cook them in your slow cooker, but these couple of dishes come out very well.

## Maria's Eggs Florentine

Our tester, Maria, came up with this recipe herself.

2 cups (225 grams) shredded cheddar cheese, divided
10 ounces (280 grams) frozen chopped spinach, thawed and drained
8 ounces (225 grams) canned mushroom, drained
1/4 cup (25 grams) chopped onion
6 eggs, beaten
1 cup (235 milliliters) heavy cream
1 teaspoon black pepper
1/2 teaspoon Italian seasoning
1/2 teaspoon garlic powder

Spray your slow cooker with nonstick cooking spray. Spread 1 cup (110 grams) of the cheese on the bottom of the slow cooker. Layer the spinach, mushrooms, and onion.

In a bowl, combine the egg, cream, pepper, Italian seasoning, and garlic powder. Pour the mixture into the slow cooker. Top with the remaining 1 cup (110 grams) cheese. Cover the slow cooker, set it to high, and let it cook for 2 hours, or until the center is set.

**YIELD:** 4 servings, each with: 568 calories, 48 g fat, 27 g protein, 10 g carbohydrate, 4 g dietary fiber, 6 g usable carbs.

# Broccoli-Bacon-Colby Quiche

This crustless quiche is wonderful, but feel free to make any quiche recipe you've got, minus the crust, in the same way. For this recipe, I use broccoli cuts that are bigger than chopped broccoli, but smaller than florets, and I think they're ideal.

2 cups (500 grams) frozen broccoli florets, thawed and coarsely chopped, or a bag of broccoli cuts

2 cups (225 grams) shredded Colby cheese

6 slices cooked bacon

4 eggs

2 cups (475 milliliters) Carb Countdown dairy beverage

1 teaspoon salt or Vege-Sal

1 teaspoon dry mustard

2 teaspoons prepared horseradish

1/4 teaspoon pepper

Spray a 1 1/2-quart glass casserole dish with nonstick cooking spray.

Put the broccoli in the bottom of the casserole dish. Spread the cheese evenly on top of the broccoli and crumble the bacon evenly over the cheese.

In a bowl, whisk together the eggs, Carb Countdown, salt or Vege-Sal, dry mustard, horseradish, and pepper and pour it over the broccoli in the casserole dish.

Place the casserole dish in your slow cooker and carefully pour water around the casserole dish to within 1" of the rim. Cover the slow cooker, set it to low, and let it cook for 4 hours.

Then turn off the slow cooker, uncover it, and let the water cool until you can remove the casserole dish without risk of scalding your fingers. Serve hot or at room temperature.

**YIELD:** 6 servings, each with: 292 calories, 21 g fat, 20 g protein, 6 g carbohydrate, 2 g dietary fiber, 4 g usable carbs.

# CHAPTER THREE

# Slow Cooker Poultry

Here you will find roughly a billion ways to fix chicken, and some ideas for turkey, too! You'll notice that many (but not all) of these recipes call for the poultry to be skinless. This is because the skin usually doesn't end up very tasty or interesting when moist-cooked as it is in a slow cooker.

I've often specified light meat or dark meat—breasts versus thighs. This is just what appealed to me. Feel free to use whichever you like best, or what's on sale. Often it's cheapest to buy a whole cut-up chicken and strip the skin off yourself at home. That's fine, too—just remove any obvious globs of fat, so your sauce doesn't end up greasy.

# Chicken Burritos

Wow. This is easy, delicious, low-carb, low-calorie, and reheats easily. What more do you want from a recipe?

2 1/2 pounds (1.25 kilograms) boneless, skinless chicken thighs

5 cloves garlic, crushed

2 tablespoons (15 grams) chili powder

2 tablespoons (28 milliliters) olive oil

2 tablespoons (28 milliliters) lime juice

1 teaspoon salt

1 large jalapeño, minced, or 2 teaspoons canned jalapeños

12 6-inch low-carb tortillas

1 cup (70 grams) shredded lettuce

1 cup (110 grams) shredded cheddar cheese

2/3 cup (180 grams) light sour cream

3/4 cup (195 grams) salsa

1/2 cup (10 grams) chopped fresh cilantro (optional)

Place the chicken in your slow cooker.

In a bowl, mix the garlic, chili powder, oil, lime juice, salt, and jalapeño together. Pour over the chicken and stir to coat. Cover the slow cooker, set it to low, and let it cook for 10 hours. (Or cook on high for 5 hours.)

When the time's up, stir the mixture with a fork to reduce the chicken to a big pot of tasty chicken shreds. Fill each tortilla with 1/3 cup chicken and top with lettuce, cheese, 1 tablespoon sour cream, a generous tablespoon salsa, and a sprinkling of cilantro if desired. Wrap and devour!

This is a great meal for a family that has some low-carbers and some non–low-carbers, just give them regular or (preferably) whole wheat flour tortillas. The chicken keeps well in the fridge, and reheats quickly in the microwave for a fast snack. (I find that 45 seconds on 70 percent power is about right for a 1/3-cup serving.)

**YIELD:** 12 servings, each with: 225 calories, 13 g fat, 22 g protein, 14 g carbohydrate, 9 g dietary fiber, 5 g usable carbs.

# Seriously Simple Chicken Chili

The name says it all!

> 2 pounds (1 kilogram) boneless, skinless chicken breasts
>
> 16 ounce (455 gram) jar prepared salsa
>
> 1 tablespoon (7 grams) chili powder
>
> 1 teaspoon chicken bouillon concentrate
>
> 3 ounces (85 grams) shredded Monterey Jack cheese
>
> 6 tablespoons (90 grams) light sour cream

Put the chicken in your slow cooker.

In a bowl, stir together the salsa, chili powder, and bouillon, making sure the bouillon's dissolved. Pour the mixture over the chicken. Cover the slow cooker, set it to low, and let it cook for 7 to 8 hours.

When the time's up, shred the chicken with a fork. Serve topped with the cheese and sour cream.

**YIELD:** 6 servings, each with: 263 calories, 9 g fat, 39 g protein, 6 g carbohydrate, 2 g dietary fiber, 4 g usable carbs.

# Chicken Chili Verde

This repeat from *15-Minute Low-Carb Recipes* is marvelous, and it's a really nice change from the traditional beef chili.

1 1/2 pounds (700 grams) boneless, skinless chicken breasts

1 1/2 cups (390 grams) prepared salsa verde

1/2 medium onion, chopped

1 bay leaf

1/2 teaspoon pepper

1 teaspoon ground cumin

1 teaspoon minced garlic or 2 cloves garlic, crushed

1–2 tablespoons (6–12 grams) jarred, sliced jalapeño
     (I use 2 tablespoons, and it makes the chili pretty hot.)

2 teaspoons chicken bouillon concentrate

Guar or xanthan (optional)

Sour cream

Shredded Monterey Jack cheese

Chopped fresh cilantro (I use 2 tablespoons, and it makes the chili pretty hot.)

Place the chicken in your slow cooker and add the salsa verde, onion, bay leaf, pepper, cumin, garlic, jalapeños, and bouillon on top. Cover the slow cooker, set it to low, and let it cook for 9 to 10 hours.

When the time's up, shred the chicken with a fork. Stir it up, thicken the chili a little with the guar or xanthan if you think it needs it, and serve with sour cream, cheese, and cilantro on top.

YIELD: 5 servings, each with: 190 calories, 2 g fat, 32 g protein, 7 g carbohydrate, trace dietary fiber, 7 g usable carbs. (Analysis does not include garnishes.)

# Chicken Cacciatore

Here's a slow cooker version of an old favorite. It's easy, too, what I call a dump-and-go recipe.

> 6 skinless chicken leg and side quarters (about 3 lbs/1.5 kg)
>
> 2 cups (500 grams) no-sugar-added spaghetti sauce (I use Hunt's.)
>
> 8 ounces (225 grams) whole canned mushrooms, drained
>
> 2 teaspoons dried oregano
>
> 1/2 cup (50 grams) chopped onion
>
> 1 green bell pepper, diced
>
> 2 cloves garlic, crushed
>
> 1/4 cup (60 milliliters) dry red wine
>
> Guar or xanthan (optional)

Simply put everything except the guar or xanthan in your slow cooker and stir it up to combine. Cover the slow cooker, set it to low, and let it cook for 7 hours.

When the time's up, remove the chicken with tongs and put it in a big serving bowl. Thicken the sauce up a little with the guar or xanthan if it needs it and ladle the sauce over the chicken.

If you like, you can serve this over Cauli-Rice (page 239), spaghetti squash, or even low-carb pasta, but I'd probably eat it as is.

**YIELD:** 6 servings, each with: 293 calories, 8 g fat, 42 g protein, 11 g carbohydrate, 4 g dietary fiber, 7 g usable carbs.

# Chicken Paprikash

Hungarian decadence! Feel free to use full-fat sour cream in this sumptuous gravy if you prefer. Or you could use plain yogurt, just drain off any watery whey first.

1/2 cup (50 grams) chopped onion

1 tablespoon (14 grams) butter

1 tablespoon (14 milliliters) oil

3 pounds (1.5 kilograms) chicken thighs

1/2 cup (120 milliliters) chicken broth

1/4 cup (60 milliliters) dry white wine

1 1/2 tablespoons (24 grams) tomato paste

1 teaspoon chicken bouillon concentrate

1 1/2 tablespoons (10 grams) paprika

1/2 teaspoon caraway seeds

1/4 teaspoon pepper

1/2 cup (120 grams) light sour cream

Guar or xanthan (optional)

In a big, heavy skillet, sauté the onion in the butter and oil over medium-low heat, until it's just golden. Transfer it to your slow cooker. Add the chicken to the skillet, turn the heat up to medium, and brown the chicken all over. Transfer it to the slow cooker, too.

Pour off the fat from the skillet and pour in the broth and wine. Stir it around to dissolve the tasty brown stuff stuck to the skillet, then stir in the tomato paste and bouillon. When those are dissolved, pour the liquid over the chicken.

Sprinkle the paprika, caraway seeds, and pepper over the chicken. Cover the slow cooker, set it to low, and let it cook for 6 hours.

When the time's up, remove the chicken with tongs or a slotted spoon and put it on a platter. Whisk the sour cream into the liquid in the slow cooker and thicken it further with guar or xanthan if desired. Serve the sauce with the chicken.

Don't forget to serve this with Fauxtatoes (see recipe page 239) to ladle this beautiful gravy onto!

**YIELD:** 5 servings, each with: 537 calories, 39 g fat, 39 g protein, 5 g carbohydrate, 1 g dietary fiber, 4 g usable carbs.

# Curried Chicken with Coconut Milk

The day I first made this, my cleaning crew was here, and they couldn't stop talking about how great it smelled. It tastes even better! Find coconut milk in the Asian section of big grocery stores or at Asian markets. It comes in regular or light, and they generally have the same carb count, so choose whichever you prefer.

3 pounds (1.5 kilograms) skinless chicken thighs

1/2 cup (50 grams) chopped onion

2 cloves garlic, crushed

1 1/2 tablespoons (9 grams) curry powder

1 cup (235 milliliters) coconut milk

1 teaspoon chicken bouillon concentrate

Guar or xanthan

Put the chicken in your slow cooker. Place the onion and garlic over it.

In a bowl, mix together the curry powder, coconut milk, and bouillon. Pour the mixture over the chicken and vegetables in the slow cooker. Cover the slow cooker, set it to low, and let it cook for 6 hours.

When the time's up, remove the chicken and put it on a platter. Thicken the sauce to a gravy consistency with guar or xanthan.

You'll want to serve this with Cauli-Rice (see recipe page 239) to soak up the extra curry sauce. It's too good to miss!

**YIELD:** 5 servings, each with: 310 calories, 18 g fat, 32 g protein, 6 g carbohydrate, 2 g dietary fiber, 4 g usable carbs.

# Chicken Vindaloo

I made this at a local campground over Memorial Day Weekend, and it was a huge hit with fellow campers. It's exotic and wonderful.

6 pounds (3 kilograms) boneless, skinless chicken thighs

1 medium onion, chopped

5 cloves garlic, crushed

1/4 cup (32 grams) grated ginger root

4 teaspoons Garam Masala (see recipe page 236) or purchased garam masala

1 teaspoon ground turmeric

1/4 cup (60 milliliters) lime juice

1/4 cup (60 milliliters) rice vinegar

1/2 cup (120 milliliters) chicken broth

1 teaspoon salt

Put the chicken, onion, and garlic in your slow cooker.

In a bowl, stir together the ginger, garam masala, turmeric, lime juice, vinegar, broth, and salt. Pour the mixture over the chicken. Cover the slow cooker, set it to low, and let it cook for 6 to 7 hours.

Serve with Slow Cooker Chutney (see recipe page 208).

**YIELD:** 12 servings, each with: 295 calories, 10 g fat, 46 g protein, 2 g carbohydrate, trace dietary fiber, 2 g usable carbs.

# Chicken with Raspberry-Chipotle Sauce

Oh, my, is this wonderful. My only regret about this recipe is that the Raspberry-Chipotle Sauce loses its brilliant ruby color during the long, slow cooking. But the flavor definitely remains. Consider using this simple sauce uncooked as a condiment on roasted poultry or pork. If you can't find raspberry syrup at a local coffee joint, you can order it online.

- 3 pounds (1.5 kilograms) chicken
- 6 teaspoons adobo seasoning
- 2 tablespoons (28 milliliters) oil
- 1 cup (110 grams) raspberries
- 1/4 cup (60 milliliters) raspberry-flavored sugar-free coffee flavoring syrup (I used Atkins brand, but Da Vinci would be fine, too.)
- 1 chipotle chile canned in adobo sauce
- 1 tablespoon (14 milliliters) white wine vinegar
- 1/4 cup (5 grams) chopped fresh cilantro (optional)

Sprinkle the chicken all over with the adobo seasoning.

In a big, heavy skillet, heat the oil over medium-high heat, then brown the chicken all over. Transfer the chicken to your slow cooker.

In a blender or food processor with the S-blade in place, combine the raspberries, raspberry-flavored coffee syrup, chipotle, and vinegar. Process till smooth. Pour the mixture evenly over the chicken. Cover the slow cooker, set it to low, and let it cook for 6 hours.

Stir the sauce before serving it over the chicken. Sprinkle a little cilantro over each piece of chicken, if desired.

**YIELD:** 5 servings, each with: 492 calories, 36 g fat, 35 g protein, 5 g carbohydrate, 2 g dietary fiber, 3 g usable carbs.

# Chicken Stew

This dish is a nice change from the usual beef stew. It's light, flavorful, and your whole meal in one pot.

2 tablespoons (28 milliliters) olive oil

1 1/2 pounds (700 grams) boneless, skinless chicken thighs, cut into 1" cubes

8 ounces (225 grams) sliced mushrooms

1 medium onion, sliced

3 cups (340 grams) zucchini slices

4 cloves garlic, crushed

14 ounces (400 grams) canned tomato wedges

3/4 cup (175 milliliters) chicken broth

1 teaspoon chicken bouillon concentrate

1 tablespoon (4 grams) poultry seasoning

Guar or xanthan

In a big, heavy skillet, heat 1 tablespoon of the oil. Brown the chicken until it is golden all over. Transfer the chicken to your slow cooker.

Heat the remaining 1 tablespoon of oil in the skillet and sauté the mushrooms, onion, and zucchini until the mushrooms change color and the onions are translucent. Transfer them to the slow cooker, too. Add the garlic and tomatoes to the slow cooker.

Put the broth and bouillon in the skillet and stir them around to dissolve any flavorful bits sticking to the skillet. Pour into the slow cooker. Sprinkle the poultry seasoning over the mixture. Cover the slow cooker, set it to low, and let it cook for 4 to 5 hours.

When the time's up, thicken the liquid in the slow cooker with guar or xanthan.

YIELD: 6 servings, each with: 159 calories, 8 g fat, 11 g protein, 12 g carbohydrate, 2 g dietary fiber, 10 g usable carbs.

# Chicken with Root Vegetables, Cabbage, and Herbs

I think of this as being a sort of French Country dish. Of course, I've never been to the French countryside, so what do I know? It's good, though, and you don't need another darned thing with it.

5 pounds (2.5 kilograms) chicken
1 1/2 tablespoons (21 milliliters) olive oil
1 1/2 tablespoons (21 grams) butter
2 medium turnips, cut into 1/2" cubes
2 medium carrots, cut into 1/2" slices
1 medium onion, cut into 1/4" half-rounds
1 head cabbage
4 cloves garlic, crushed
1/2 teaspoon dried rosemary
1/2 teaspoon dried thyme
1/2 teaspoon dried basil
2 bay leaves, crumbled

In a big, heavy skillet, brown the chicken on both sides in the oil and butter over medium-high heat.

When the chicken is browned all over, remove it to a plate and reserve. Some extra fat will have accumulated in the skillet, pour off all but a couple of tablespoons, then add the turnips, carrots, and onion. Sauté them, scraping the tasty brown bits off the bottom of the skillet as you stir, until they're getting a touch of gold, too.

Transfer the sautéed vegetables to your slow cooker.

Cut the cabbage into eighths and put it on top of the vegetables. Arrange the chicken on top of the cabbage. Sprinkle the garlic over the chicken and vegetables, making sure some ends up on the chicken and some down among the vegetables. Sprinkle the rosemary, thyme, basil, and bay leaves into the slow cooker, making sure some gets down into the vegetables. Season with salt and pepper. Cover the slow cooker, set it to low, and let it cook for 6 to 7 hours.

**YIELD:** 8 servings, each with: 510 calories, 37 g fat, 36 g protein, 6 g carbohydrate, 2 g dietary fiber, 4 g usable carbs.

# ☐ Citrus Spice Chicken

Sunshiny citrus flavor! Another dump-and-go recipe.

1/3 cup (78 milliliters) lemon juice

2 tablespoons (3 grams) Splenda

1/2 teaspoon orange extract

1/2 cup (120 grams) Dana's No-Sugar Ketchup (see recipe page 228)
   or purchased low-carb ketchup

2 tablespoons (40 grams) low-sugar orange marmalade

1/2 teaspoon ground cinnamon

1/2 teaspoon ground allspice

1/8 teaspoon ground cloves

1/4 teaspoon cayenne

3 pounds (1.5 kilograms) skinless chicken thighs

In a bowl, stir together the lemon juice, Splenda, orange extract, ketchup, marmalade, cinnamon, allspice, cloves, and cayenne.

Put the chicken in your slow cooker and pour the sauce over it. Cover the slow cooker, set it to low, and let it cook for 6 hours.

Serve with Cauli-Rice (see recipe page 239).

YIELD: 5 servings, each with: 191 calories, 6 g fat, 31 g protein, 2 g carbohydrate, trace dietary fiber, 2 g usable carbs.

# Italian Chicken and Vegetables

1/2 head cabbage, cut in wedges

1 medium onion, sliced

8 ounces (225 grams) sliced mushrooms

2 pounds (1 kilogram) skinless chicken breasts

2 pounds (1 kilogram) skinless chicken thighs

2 cups (500 grams) no-sugar-added spaghetti sauce (I use Hunt's.)

Guar or xanthan (optional)

Grated Parmesan cheese

Put the cabbage, onion, and mushrooms in your slow cooker. Place the chicken on top of the vegetables. Pour the spaghetti sauce over the top.

Cover the slow cooker, set it to low, and let it cook for 6 hours. Thicken the sauce with guar or xanthan if needed and serve with Parmesan cheese.

**YIELD:** 6 servings, each with: 254 calories, 5 g fat, 46 g protein, 4 g carbohydrate, 1 g dietary fiber, 3 g usable carbs.

# Lemon Chicken

3 pounds (1.5 kilogram) skinless chicken thighs

2 tablespoons (28 grams) butter

1 teaspoon dried oregano

1/2 teaspoon seasoned salt

1/4 teaspoon pepper

1/4 cup (60 milliliters) chicken broth

3 tablespoons (45 milliliters) lemon juice

2 cloves garlic, crushed

2 tablespoons (8 grams) chopped fresh parsley

1 teaspoon chicken bouillon concentrate

Guar or xanthan

In a big, heavy skillet, brown the chicken in the butter over medium-high heat.

In a bowl, mix together the oregano, seasoned salt, and pepper. When the chicken is golden, sprinkle the spice mixture over it. Transfer the chicken to your slow cooker.

Pour the broth and lemon juice in the skillet, stirring around to deglaze the pan. Add the garlic, parsley, and bouillon. Stir until the bouillon dissolves. Pour into the slow cooker.

Cover the slow cooker, set it to low, and let it cook for 4 to 5 hours. When the chicken is tender, remove it from the slow cooker. Thicken the sauce a bit with guar or xanthan. Serve the sauce with the chicken.

This dish goes well with Cauli-Rice (see recipe page 239).

**YIELD:** 6 servings, each with: 200 calories, 9 g fat, 26 g protein, 2 g carbohydrate, 1 g dietary fiber, 1 g usable carbs.

# Chicken with Thyme and Artichokes

This is sort of classic, yet very little work.

1 1/2 pounds (700 grams) boneless, skinless chicken thighs

2 tablespoons (28 milliliters) olive oil

1/2 cup (120 milliliters) dry white wine

1 tablespoon (14 milliliters) lemon juice

1 teaspoon chicken bouillon concentrate

2 teaspoons dried thyme

1 clove garlic, crushed

1/4 teaspoon pepper

13 ounces (370 grams) canned artichoke hearts, drained

Guar or xanthan

In a big, heavy skillet, brown the chicken in the oil over medium-high heat until golden on both sides. Transfer to your slow cooker.

In a bowl, stir together the wine, lemon juice, bouillon, thyme, garlic, and pepper. Pour the mixture over the chicken. Place the artichokes on top. Cover the slow cooker, set it to low, and let it cook for 6 hours.

Scoop out the chicken and artichokes with a slotted spoon. Thicken the liquid left in the pot with just enough guar or xanthan to make it the thickness of half-and-half.

Serve the chicken and artichokes, plus the sauce, over Cauli-Rice (see recipe page 239).

**YIELD:** 4 servings, each with: 314 calories, 10 g fat, 42 g protein, 7 g carbohydrate, trace dietary fiber, 7 g usable carbs.

# Lemon–White Wine–Tarragon Chicken

This is similar to the previous recipe, except, of course, that tarragon is very different from thyme and there are no artichokes.

3 pounds (1.5 kilograms) skinless chicken thighs

1/2 cup (120 milliliters) dry white wine

1/2 cup (120 milliliter) lemon juice

1 teaspoon Splenda

1 tablespoon (2 grams) dried tarragon

1/2 teaspoon pepper

1 teaspoon chicken bouillon concentrate

Guar or xanthan

Put the chicken in your slow cooker.

In a bowl, mix together the wine, lemon juice, Splenda, tarragon, pepper, and bouillon, stirring until the bouillon dissolves. Pour the mixture over the chicken. Cover the slow cooker, set it to low, and let it cook for 6 hours.

Remove the chicken to serving plates and thicken the remaining liquid with guar or xanthan to achieve the texture of cream.

**YIELD:** 6 servings, each with: 176 calories, 5 g fat, 26 g protein, 3 g carbohydrate, trace dietary fiber, 3 g usable carbs.

# Mom's 1960s Chicken, Redux

Back in the 1960s my mom would make a dish for company with chicken breasts, wrapped in bacon, laid on a layer of chipped beef, topped with a sauce made of sour cream and cream of mushroom soup. It tasted far more sophisticated than it sounds and never failed to draw raves from dinner party guests. This is my attempt to de-carb and slow-cooker-ize the same dish — without the carb-filled cream of mushroom soup.

2 1/4 ounces (62 grams) dried beef slices (aka "chipped beef")

6 slices bacon

2 pounds (1 kilogram) boneless, skinless chicken breasts

1 cup (100 grams) sliced mushrooms

1 tablespoon (14 grams) butter

1 cup (235 milliliters) heavy cream

1 teaspoon beef bouillon concentrate

1 pinch onion powder

1 pinch celery salt

1/4 teaspoon pepper

Guar or xanthan

1 cup (230 grams) sour cream

Paprika

Line the bottom of your slow cooker with the dried beef.

Place the bacon in a glass pie plate or on a microwave bacon rack and microwave for 3 to 4 minutes on high. Drain the bacon and reserve. (What you're doing here is cooking some of the grease off of the bacon, without cooking it crisp.)

Cut the chicken into 6 servings. Wrap each piece of chicken in a slice of bacon and place it in the slow cooker on top of the dried beef.

In a big, heavy skillet, sauté the mushrooms in the butter until they're soft. Add the cream and bouillon and stir until the bouillon dissolves. Stir in the onion powder, celery salt, and pepper, then thicken with guar or xanthan until the mixture reaches a gravy consistency. Stir in the sour cream.

Spoon this mixture over the chicken breasts and sprinkle with a little paprika. Cover the slow cooker, set it to low, and let it cook for 5 to 6 hours.

To serve, scoop up some of the dried beef and sauce with each bacon-wrapped piece of chicken.

**YIELD:** 6 servings, each with: 472 calories, 32 g fat, 41 g protein, 4 g carbohydrate, trace dietary fiber, 4 g usable carbs.

# 🍲 Slow Cooker Chicken Mole

Chicken mole is the national dish of Mexico, and I'm crazy about it. On my honeymoon in Mexico, I bought a container of chicken mole at the deli at the local grocery store and kept it in the hotel room fridge to heat up in the microwave! Here's a slow cooker version.

14 1/2 ounces (411 grams) canned tomatoes with green chiles

1/2 cup (50 grams) chopped onion

1/4 cup (30 grams) slivered almonds, toasted

3 cloves garlic, crushed

3 tablespoons (17 grams) unsweetened cocoa powder

2 tablespoons (35 grams) raisins

1 tablespoon (7 grams) sesame seeds

1 tablespoon (1.5 grams) Splenda

1/4 teaspoon ground cinnamon

1/4 teaspoon ground nutmeg

1/4 teaspoon ground coriander

1/4 teaspoon salt

3 pounds (1.5 kilograms) skinless chicken thighs

Guar or xanthan

2 tablespoons (15 grams) slivered almonds, toasted

Put the tomatoes, onion, 1/4 cup almonds, garlic, cocoa powder, raisins, sesame seeds, Splenda, cinnamon, nutmeg, coriander, and salt in a blender or food processor and puree coarsely.

Place the chicken in your slow cooker. Pour the sauce over it. Cover the slow cooker, set it to low, and let it cook for 9 to 10 hours.

Remove the chicken from the slow cooker with tongs. Thicken the sauce to taste with guar or xanthan. Serve the sauce over the chicken. Top with the 2 tablespoons almonds.

**YIELD:** 8 servings, each with: 284 calories, 12 g fat, 37 g protein, 8 g carbohydrate, 2 g dietary fiber, 6 g usable carbs.

# Mediterranean Chicken

This recipe, bursting with classic Mediterranean flavors, originally appeared in *500 More Low-Carb Recipes*.

 8 ounces (225 grams) sliced mushrooms
 14 1/2 ounces (411 grams) canned tomatoes
 6 ounces (170 grams) canned artichoke hearts
 2 1/2 ounces (70 grams) sliced black olives
 3 pounds (1.5 kilograms) skinless chicken thighs
 1 tablespoon (4 grams) Italian seasoning
 3/4 cup (175 milliliters) chicken broth
 1 teaspoon chicken bouillon concentrate
 1/4 cup (60 milliliters) dry white wine
 Guar or xanthan

Put the mushrooms, tomatoes, artichokes, and olives in your slow cooker. Place the chicken on top.

In a bowl, mix together the Italian seasoning, broth, bouillon, and wine. Pour the sauce over the chicken and vegetables. Cover the slow cooker, set it to low, and let it cook for 7 hours.

When the time's up, thicken the juices a bit with guar or xanthan.

**YIELD:** 6 servings, each with: 215 calories, 7 g fat, 28 g protein, 8 g carbohydrate, 2 g dietary fiber, 6 g usable carbs.

#  Orange Teriyaki Chicken

This has been officially rated "Very Easy, Very Good!"

16 ounces (455 grams) frozen Oriental vegetable mixture, unthawed

2 pounds (1 kilogram) boneless, skinless chicken breasts, cubed

3/4 cup (175 milliliters) chicken broth

2 tablespoons (35 grams) Low-Carb Teriyaki Sauce (see recipe page 233)

    or purchased low-carb teriyaki sauce

1 teaspoon chicken bouillon concentrate

1 tablespoon (20 grams) low-sugar orange marmalade

1/4 teaspoon orange extract

2 tablespoons (28 milliliters) lemon juice

1 teaspoon Splenda

1 teaspoon dry mustard

1/2 teaspoon ground ginger

Guar or xanthan

Pour the vegetables into your slow cooker. Place the chicken on top.

In a bowl, combine the broth, teriyaki sauce, bouillon, marmalade, orange extract, lemon juice, Splenda, dry mustard, and ginger, stirring well. Pour the mixture over the chicken and veggies. Cover the slower cooker, set it to low, and let it cook for 4 to 5 hours.

Before serving, thicken the sauce a bit with guar or xanthan.

Serve over Cauli-Rice (see recipe page 239) if desired. Or for the carbivores you can serve it over brown rice, lo mein noodles, or plain old spaghetti.

**YIELD:** 6 servings, each with: 222 calories, 4 g fat, 36 g protein, 7 g carbohydrate, 2 g dietary fiber, 5 g usable carbs.

# Thai Chicken Bowls

This was a big hit with Maria's family!

8 boneless, skinless, boneless chicken thighs, cubed (a little over 2 1/4 lbs/1 kg)

2 cloves garlic, crushed

1/2 cup (50 grams) chopped onion

2 stalks celery, sliced

2 teaspoons grated ginger root

1 teaspoon five-spice powder

1/2 teaspoon salt

1 tablespoon (14 milliliters) lemon juice

1 teaspoon hot sauce (optional)

28 ounces (850 milliliters) chicken broth

1 head cauliflower

Guar or xanthan

6 tablespoons (35 grams) sliced scallions

6 tablespoons (7 grams) chopped cilantro

Place the chicken in your slow cooker. Top with the garlic, onion, celery, ginger, five-spice powder, salt, and lemon juice.

In a bowl, combine the hot sauce, if using, with the broth and pour it into the slow cooker. Cover the slow cooker, set it to low, and let it cook for 5 to 6 hours.

Okay, it's almost supper time. Run your cauliflower through the shredding blade of your food processor to make Cauli-Rice. Put your Cauli-Rice in a microwaveable casserole with a lid, add a couple of tablespoons of water, cover, and microwave on high for 6 minutes.

Thicken up the sauce in the slow cooker with a little guar or xanthan to about the texture of heavy cream.

Okay, Cauli-Rice is done! Uncover it immediately, drain, and divide it into 6 bowls. Divide the chicken mixture, ladling it over the Cauli-Rice. Top with the scallions and cilantro.

**YIELD:** 6 servings, each with: 138 calories, 4 g fat, 20 g protein, 4 g carbohydrate, 1 g dietary fiber, 3 g usable carbs.

# Thai Hot Pot

This recipe takes a few more steps than some, but the results are worth it! If you can't get Southeast Asian fish sauce, you can substitute soy sauce.

1 1/2 pounds (700 grams) boneless, skinless chicken thighs

1 medium carrot, sliced

1 medium onion, sliced

1 clove garlic, crushed

14 ounces (425 milliliters) coconut milk

1 tablespoon (8 grams) grated ginger root

2 tablespoons (35 grams) fish sauce (nam pla or nuoc mam) or soy sauce

1 tablespoon (14 milliliters) lime juice

2 teaspoons Splenda

1/2 teaspoon hot sauce

1/3 cup (90 grams) natural peanut butter

1 pound (455 grams) shrimp, shelled

1 cup (75 grams) fresh snow pea pods, cut into 1/2" pieces

Guar or xanthan

6 cups (720 grams) Cauli-Rice (see recipe page 239)

1/3 cup (60 grams) chopped peanuts

Put the chicken in your slow cooker and add the carrot, onion, and garlic.

In a blender, combine the coconut milk, ginger, fish sauce or soy sauce, lime juice, Splenda, hot sauce, and peanut butter and blend until smooth. Pour the sauce over the chicken and vegetables, using a rubber scraper to make sure you get all of it! Cover the slow cooker, set it to low, and let it cook for 8 hours.

Stir in the shrimp and snow peas, re-cover the slow cooker, and turn it up to high. Cook for 10 minutes, or until the shrimp are pink through.

Thicken the sauce slightly with guar or xanthan. Serve over the Cauli-Rice (or brown rice, for the carb-eaters.) Top each serving with the peanuts.

**YIELD:** 6 servings, each with: 480 calories, 32 g fat, 33 g protein, 19 g carbohydrate, 7 g dietary fiber, 12 g usable carbs.

# Yassa

This chicken stew comes from Senegal. Traditionally it is quite hot, so feel free to increase the cayenne if you like!

> 3 large onions, thinly sliced
> 6 cloves garlic, crushed
> 1/2 cup (120 milliliters) lemon juice
> 1 1/2 teaspoons salt
> 1/2 teaspoon cayenne, or more to taste
> 6 pounds (3 kilograms) chicken, cut up
> 1/4 cup (60 milliliters) oil
> 8 cups (960 grams) Cauli-Rice (see recipe page 239)

In your slow cooker, combine the onions, garlic, lemon juice, salt, and cayenne. Add the chicken and toss, so that all the chicken comes in contact with the seasonings. Cover your slow cooker and refrigerate overnight. (It's a good idea to stir this a few times if you think of it, though I don't expect you to get up in the middle of the night to do it!)

Using tongs, remove the chicken from the marinade. Pat it dry with paper towels and set it aside. Transfer the marinade to your slow cooker.

In a big, heavy skillet, heat the oil over medium-high heat. Place the chicken skin side down, and cook it until the skin is browned. (You'll need to do this in batches, unless your skillet is a lot bigger than mine!) Don't bother browning the other side of the chicken.

Transfer the chicken back to the slow cooker with the marinade. Cover the slow cooker, set it to low, and let it cook for 5 to 6 hours.

Remove the chicken from the slow cooker with tongs. Put the chicken on a platter, cover it with foil, and put it in a warm place.

Ladle the onions and liquid out of the slow cooker into the skillet and turn the heat to high. Boil this hard, stirring often, until most of the liquid has evaporated. (You want the volume reduced by more than half.) Serve the chicken, onions, and sauce over the Cauli-Rice.

**YIELD:** 8 servings, each with: 638 calories, 46 g fat, 45 g protein, 11 g carbohydrate, 3 g dietary fiber, 8 g usable carbs.

# Southwestern Barbecue

This is incredibly popular, for something so easy!

 1/2 cup (125 grams) tomato sauce
 1 tablespoon (1.5 grams) Splenda
 1 1/2 tablespoons (9 grams) canned, sliced jalapeños
 2 tablespoons (28 milliliters) lime juice
 1/8 teaspoon blackstrap molasses
 1 teaspoon ground cumin
 1/4 teaspoon red pepper flakes
 4 pounds (2 kilograms) skinless chicken thighs

Combine everything except for the chicken in your slow cooker and stir well. Place the chicken in the sauce, meaty side down. Cover the slow cooker, set it to low, and let it cook for 6 hours.

Serve the chicken with the sauce spooned over it.

**YIELD:** 6 servings, each with: 215 calories, 7 g fat, 34 g protein, 2 g carbohydrate, trace dietary fiber, 2 g usable carbs.

# Chicken and Dumplings

This takes some work, but boy, is it comfort food. You could make this with leftover turkey instead if you prefer. If you do that, put the cubed, cooked turkey in about 5 to 6 hours into the initial cooking time.

2 medium carrots, sliced

1 medium onion, chunked

2 medium turnips, cut into 1/2" cubes

1 1/2 cups (225 grams) frozen green beans, cross-cut

8 ounces (225 grams) sliced mushrooms

1 1/2 pounds (700 grams) boneless, skinless chicken thighs, cut into 1" cubes

1 1/2 cups (355 milliliters) chicken broth

1 teaspoon poultry seasoning

3 teaspoons chicken bouillon concentrate

1/2 cup (120 milliliters) heavy cream

Guar or xanthan

Dumplings (see recipe on next page)

In your slow cooker, combine the carrots, onion, turnips, green beans, mushrooms, and chicken.

In a bowl, mix together the broth, poultry seasoning, and bouillon. Pour the mixture over the chicken and vegetables. Cover the slow cooker, set it to low, and let it cook for 6 to 7 hours.

When the time's up, stir in the cream and thicken the gravy to a nice consistency with guar or xanthan. Add salt and pepper to taste. Re-cover the slow cooker and turn it to high.

While the slow cooker is heating up (it'll take at least 30 minutes), make your Dumplings, stopping before you add the liquid. Wait until the gravy in the slow cooker is boiling. Then stir in the buttermilk and drop the biscuit dough by spoonfuls over the surface of the chicken and gravy. Re-cover the slow cooker and let it cook for another 25 to 30 minutes.

**YIELD:** 8 servings, each with: 417 calories, 25 g fat, 36 g protein, 14 g carbohydrate, 4 g dietary fiber, 10 g usable carbs. (Calculations include the Dumplings.)

# Dumplings

Feel free to use this with other meat-and-gravy dishes if you like! (These instructions require gravy to boil the Dumplings in.)

3/4 cup (110 grams) ground almonds, or "almond meal"

1/2 cup (120 grams) rice protein powder (Get this at your health food store. If they don't have it, they can order it. I use NutriBiotic brand.)

1/4 cup (28 grams) wheat gluten

2 tablespoons (28 grams) butter

2 tablespoons (28 milliliters) coconut oil

1/2 teaspoon salt

2 teaspoons baking powder

1/2 teaspoon baking soda

3/4 cup (175 milliliters) buttermilk

Put everything but the buttermilk into your food processor with the S-blade in place. Pulse the food processor to cut in the butter. (You want it evenly distributed in the dry ingredients.) Dump this mixture into a mixing bowl.

Check to make sure your gravy is boiling. (If it isn't, have a quick cup of tea until it is.) Now pour the buttermilk into the dry ingredients and stir it in with a few swift strokes. (Don't over-mix; you just want to make sure everything's evenly damp.) This will make a soft dough. Drop by spoonfuls over the boiling gravy, cover the pot, and let it cook for 25 to 30 minutes.

**NOTE:** Grind 3/4 cup almonds to cormeal-like consistency, or use almond meal.

**YIELD:** 12 servings, each with: 153 calories, 10 g fat, 14 g protein, 4 g carbohydrate, 1 g dietary fiber, 3 g usable carbs.

# Chicken in Creamy Horseradish Sauce

Don't think that just because this has horseradish it's really strong. The sauce is mellow, subtle, and family-friendly.

4 pounds (2 kilograms) cut-up chicken
1 tablespoon (14 grams) butter
1 tablespoon (14 milliliters) olive oil
3/4 cup (175 milliliters) chicken broth
1 1/2 teaspoons chicken bouillon concentrate
1 tablespoon (15 grams) prepared horseradish
4 ounces (115 grams) cream cheese, cut into chunks
1/4 cup (60 milliliters) heavy cream
Guar or xanthan (optional)

In a big, heavy skillet, brown the chicken in the butter and oil over medium-high heat. Transfer the chicken to your slow cooker.

In a bowl, stir together the broth, bouillon, and horseradish. Pour the mixture over the chicken. Cover the slow cooker, set it to low, and let it cook for 6 hours.

When the time's up, remove the chicken with tongs and put it on a platter. Melt the cream cheese into the sauce in the slow cooker. Stir in the cream. Thicken the sauce with guar or xanthan if you think it needs it. Add salt and pepper to taste.

I think this would be good with Fauxtatoes (see recipe page 239) and green beans.

**YIELD:** 8 servings, each with: 442 calories, 34 g fat, 30 g protein, 1 g carbohydrate, trace dietary fiber, 1 g usable carbs.

# Chicken in Creamy Orange Sauce

4 pounds (2 kilograms) skinless chicken thighs

3 tablespoons (45 milliliters) oil

3 tablespoons (45 milliliters) brandy

1/2 cup (120 milliliters) white wine vinegar

1/2 cup (120 milliliters) lemon juice

1/2 teaspoon orange extract

1 teaspoon grated orange rind

1/3 cup (8 grams) Splenda

8 scallions, sliced

6 ounces (170 grams) light cream cheese, cut into chunks

Guar or xanthan (optional)

In a big, heavy skillet, brown the chicken in the oil over medium-high heat. Transfer the chicken to your slow cooker.

In a bowl, stir together the brandy, vinegar, lemon juice, orange extract, and Splenda. Pour the mixture over chicken. Cover the slow cooker, set it to low, and let it cook for 6 hours.

When the time's up, transfer the chicken to a platter. Add the scallions to the liquid in the slow cooker, then add the cream cheese and stir till it's melted. Thicken with guar or xanthan if you think it needs it. Add salt and pepper to taste. Serve the sauce over the chicken.

Cauli-Rice (see recipe page 239) in one form or another is the natural side dish with this. Add a big green salad, and there's supper!

**YIELD:** 8 servings, each with: 359 calories, 20 g fat, 35 g protein, 5 g carbohydrate, trace dietary fiber, 5 g usable carbs.

# Tuscan Chicken

This is fabulous Italian chicken!

4 pounds (2 kilograms) skinless chicken thighs

1 tablespoon (14 milliliters) olive oil

1/2 cup (50 grams) chopped onion

1 red bell pepper, cut into strips

1 green bell pepper, cut into strips

15 ounces (425 grams) canned black soybeans, drained

14 1/2 ounces (411 grams) canned crushed tomatoes

1/2 cup (120 milliliters) dry white wine

1 teaspoon dried oregano

1 clove garlic, crushed

1 teaspoon chicken bouillon concentrate

In a big, heavy skillet, brown the chicken in the oil over medium-high heat.

Meanwhile, put the onion, peppers, and soybeans in your slow cooker. Place the chicken on top of the vegetables and beans.

In a bowl, stir together the tomatoes, wine, oregano, garlic, and bouillon. Pour the mixture over the chicken. Cover the slow cooker, set it to low, and let it cook for 6 to 7 hours. Add salt and pepper to taste.

YIELD: 8 servings, each with: 258 calories, 9 g fat, 31 g protein, 10 g carbohydrate, 5 g dietary fiber, 5 g usable carbs.

#  "I've Got a Life" Chicken

This recipe from *15-Minute Low-Carb Recipes* is remarkably good. It's sweet, tangy, and fruity.

3–3 1/2 pounds (1.5–2 kilograms) bone-in chicken parts
    (I use legs and thighs, but a whole cut-up chicken would work great.)
8 ounces (225 grams) sliced mushrooms
3 tablespoons (45 milliliters) orange juice
Grated zest of one orange
1 tablespoon (14 milliliters) chicken bouillon concentrate
1/2 teaspoon pepper
8 ounces (225 grams) canned tomato sauce
2 tablespoons (28 milliliters) soy sauce
2 tablespoons (3 grams) Splenda
1/2 teaspoon blackstrap molasses
2 teaspoons minced garlic or 4 cloves garlic, crushed
1 teaspoon dried thyme
Guar or xanthan

Remove the skin and any big lumps of fat from the chicken and place it in your slow cooker. (You can save time by buying chicken with the skin already removed, but it's more expensive.) Place the mushrooms on top.

In a bowl, mix together the orange juice, orange zest, bouillon, pepper, tomato sauce, soy sauce, Splenda, molasses, garlic, and thyme. Pour the mixture on top of the chicken and mushrooms. Cover the slow cooker, set it to low, and let it cook for 5 to 6 hours.

When the time's up, remove the chicken and put it on a platter. Use the guar or xanthan to thicken up the sauce in the slow cooker and serve the sauce with the chicken.

**YIELD:** 6 servings, each with: 424 calories, 27 g fat, 35 g protein, 7 g carbohydrate, 1 g dietary fiber, 6 g usable carbs. (This analysis assumes that you eat all of the gravy.)

# Slow Cooker Brewery Chicken and Vegetables

There are plenty of vegetables in here, so you don't need a thing with it, except maybe some bread for the carb-eaters in the family. And the gravy comes out a beautiful color!

8 ounces (225 grams) turnips (two turnips roughly the size of tennis balls), peeled and cut into chunks

2 stalks celery, sliced

1 medium carrot, sliced

1/2 medium onion, sliced

1 tablespoon (14 milliliters) chicken bouillon concentrate

2 1/2–3 pounds (1.25–1.5 kilograms) cut-up chicken

(I use leg and thigh quarters, cut apart at the joints.)

12 ounces (355 milliliters) light beer

14 1/2 ounces (411 grams) canned tomatoes with green chiles

Guar or xanthan (optional)

Put the turnips, celery, carrot, onion, bouillon, and chicken in your slow cooker. Pour the beer and the tomatoes over the lot. Cover the slow cooker, set it to low, and let it cook for 8 to 9 hours.

When the time's up, remove the chicken with tongs and place it on a serving platter. Then, using a slotted spoon, scoop out the vegetables. Put 1 1/2 cups (355 milliliters) of them in a blender and pile the rest on and around the chicken on the platter. Scoop out 1 1/2 to 2 cups (355 to 475 ml) of the liquid left in the slow cooker and put it in the blender with the vegetables. Puree the veggies and broth and thicken the mixture a little more with the guar or xanthan, if it seems necessary. Add salt and pepper to taste and serve as a sauce with the chicken and vegetables.

**YIELD:** 5 servings, each with: 415 calories, 26 g fat, 30 g protein, 10 g carbohydrate, 2 g dietary fiber, 8 g usable carbs.

# Slow Cooker Chicken Guadeloupe

This isn't authentically anything, but it borrows its flavors from the Creole cooking of the Caribbean.

1 cut-up broiler-fryer chicken, about 3 1/2 pounds (1.75 kilograms),
    or whatever chicken parts you prefer

1/2 medium onion, chopped

2 teaspoons ground allspice

1 teaspoon dried thyme

1/4 cup (60 milliliters) lemon juice,

14 1/2 ounces (411 grams) canned tomatoes with green chiles

1 shot (3 tablespoons/45 milliliters) dark rum

Guar or xanthan

Place the chicken, onion, allspice, thyme, lemon juice, tomatoes, and rum in your slow cooker. Cover the slow cooker, set it to low, and let it cook for 5 to 6 hours.

Remove the chicken carefully—it'll be sliding from the bone! Thicken up the sauce with guar or xanthan. Add salt and pepper to taste and serve the sauce over the chicken.

**YIELD:** 5 servings, each with: 541 calories, 36 g fat, 41 g protein, 7 g carbohydrate, 1 g dietary fiber, 6 g usable carbs.

# Sort-of-Ethiopian Chicken Stew

The slow cooker method is hardly authentic, but the flavors come from an Ethiopian recipe—except that the Ethiopians would use a lot more cayenne! Increase it if you like really hot food.

1 cut-up broiler-fryer, about 3 pounds (1.5 kilograms)

1 medium onion, chopped

1 teaspoon cayenne

1 teaspoon paprika

1/2 teaspoon pepper

1/2 teaspoon grated ginger root

2 tablespoons (28 milliliters) lemon juice

1/2 cup (120 milliliters) water

Guar or xanthan

Place the chicken, onion, cayenne, paprika, pepper, ginger, lemon juice, and water in your slow cooker. Cover the slow cooker, set it to low, and let it cook for 5 to 6 hours.

If you'd like to make this really stewlike, you can pick the meat off the bones when it's done (which will be very easy), thicken the gravy with guar or xanthan, and then stir the chicken back into the liquid. Or you can just serve the gravy over the chicken. Take your pick.

**YIELD:** 5 servings, each with: 437 calories, 31 g fat, 34 g protein, 3 g carbohydrate, 1 g dietary fiber, 2 g usable carbs.

# Cranberry-Peach Turkey Roast

This fruity sauce really wakes up the turkey roast!

3 pounds (1.5 kilograms) turkey roast

2 tablespoons (28 milliliters) oil

1/2 cup (50 grams) chopped onion

1 cup (110 grams) cranberries

1/4 cup (6 grams) Splenda

3 tablespoons (45 grams) spicy mustard

1/4 teaspoon red pepper flakes

1 peach, peeled and chopped

If your turkey roast is a Butterball like mine, it will be a boneless affair of light and dark meat rolled into an oval roast, enclosed in a net sack. Leave it in the net for cooking, so it doesn't fall apart.

In a big heavy skillet, heat the oil and brown the turkey on all sides. Transfer the turkey to the slow cooker.

In a blender or food processor with the S-blade in place, combine the onion, cranberries, Splenda, mustard, red pepper, and peach. Run it until you have a coarse puree. Pour the mixture over the turkey. Cover the slow cooker, set it to low, and let it cook for 6 to 7 hours.

Remove the turkey to a platter, stir up the sauce, and ladle it into a sauce boat to serve with the turkey. You can remove the net from the turkey before serving, if you like, but I find it easier just to use a good sharp knife to slice clear through the netting and let diners remove their own.

**YIELD:** 8 servings, each with: 255 calories, 8 g fat, 31 g protein, 4 g carbohydrate, 1 g dietary fiber, 3 g usable carbs.

# Braised Turkey Wings with Mushrooms

Turkey wings are my favorite cut of turkey for the slow cooker. They fit in easily, they come in good individual serving sizes, and, oh yeah, they taste great.

3 1/4 pounds (1.75 kilograms) turkey wings

1/4 cup (60 milliliters) olive oil

1/2 cup (120 milliliters) chicken broth

1 teaspoon chicken bouillon concentrate

1 teaspoon poultry seasoning

1 tablespoon (16 grams) tomato paste

1 cup (100 grams) sliced mushrooms

1/2 medium onion, sliced

1/2 cup (115 grams) sour cream

In a big, heavy skillet, brown the turkey all over in the oil over medium-high heat. Transfer the turkey to your slow cooker.

In a bowl, stir together the broth, bouillon, poultry seasoning, and tomato paste. Pour the mixture over the turkey. Add the mushrooms and onion. Cover the slow cooker, set it to low, and let it cook for 6 to 7 hours.

When the time's up, remove the turkey from the slow cooker with tongs. Whisk the sour cream into the sauce and serve the sauce over the turkey.

**YIELD:** 3 servings, each with: 555 calories, 40 g fat, 41 g protein, 6 g carbohydrate, 1 g dietary fiber, 5 g usable carbs.

# Ranch-E-Cue Wings

Simple!

2 pounds (1 kilogram) turkey wings

3 tablespoons (45 milliliters) olive oil

1/2 cup (120 milliliters) chicken broth

3 teaspoons ranch-style dressing mix

1/2 cup (120 grams) Dana's "Kansas City" Barbecue Sauce
(see recipe page 231) or purchased low-carb barbecue sauce

Cut the turkey wings at the joints, discarding the pointy wing tips.

In a big, heavy skillet, heat the oil and brown the turkey all over. Transfer the turkey to your slow cooker.

In a bowl, mix together the broth, dressing mix, and barbecue sauce. Pour the mixture over the wings. Cover the slow cooker, set it to low, and let it cook for 6 to 7 hours.

**YIELD:** 4 servings, each with: 246 calories, 17 g fat, 18 g protein, 5 g carbohydrate, 0 g dietary fiber, 5 g usable carbs.


# Turkey Loaf with Thai Flavors

Ground turkey is cheap, low-carb, low-calorie—and by itself just plain boring. So jazz it up by adding some Thai flavors.

2 pounds (1 kilogram) ground turkey

1 medium onion, chopped

4 1/2 ounces (130 grams) canned mushroom slices, drained

4 cloves garlic, crushed

2 tablespoons (28 milliliters) lemon juice

4 tablespoon (60 milliliters) lime juice, divided

4 teaspoons chili paste

3 tablespoons (24 grams) grated ginger root

1 1/2 tablespoons (30 grams) fish sauce

1 1/2 tablespoons (21 milliliters) soy sauce

1 1/2 teaspoons pepper

1/2 cup (60 grams) pork rind crumbs

    (Run some pork rinds through your food processor.)

1/2 cup (10 grams) chopped fresh cilantro

1/2 cup (120 grams) mayonnaise

Place the turkey in a big mixing bowl.

Place the onion, mushrooms, and garlic in a food processor. Pulse until everything is chopped medium-fine. Add it to the turkey.

Add the lemon juice, 2 tablespoons of the lime juice, the chili paste, ginger, fish sauce, soy sauce, pepper, pork rind crumbs, and cilantro to the bowl. Mix it around with clean hands until it is well blended.

Spray a rack or a collapsible-basket-type steamer with nonstick cooking spray and place it in your slow cooker. Add a cup of water under the rack. If the holes in the rack are pretty large, cover it with a sheet of foil, and pierce it all over with a fork. Take two 18" (45 centimeters) squares of foil, fold them into strips about 2" (5 centimeters) wide, and criss-cross them across the rack or steamer, running the ends up the sides of the slow cooker. (You're making a sling to help lift the meat loaf out of the slow cooker.) Place the meat mixture on the rack or steamer and form it into an evenly-domed loaf. Cover the slow cooker, set it to low, and let it cook for 6 hours.

When the time's up, use the strips of foil to gently lift the loaf out of the slow cooker and place it on a platter.

In a bowl, mix together the mayonnaise and the remaining 2 tablespoons lime juice. Cut the loaf into wedges and serve it with the lime mayonnaise.

YIELD: 8 servings, each with: 327 calories, 24 g fat, 25 g protein, 5 g carbohydrate, 1 g dietary fiber, 4 g usable carbs.

# Chipotle Turkey Legs

This dish has spicy, rich Southwestern flavor.

> 3 turkey drumsticks, about 2 pounds (1 kilogram) total
>
> 1 1/2 teaspoons cumin
>
> 1 teaspoon chili powder
>
> 1 teaspoon dried, powdered sage
>
> 1 teaspoon minced garlic or 2 cloves garlic, crushed
>
> 1/2 teaspoon red pepper flakes
>
> 1/4 teaspoon turmeric
>
> 1 or 2 canned chipotle chiles in adobo sauce, plus a couple teaspoons
>    of the sauce they come in
>
> 8 ounces (225 grams) tomato sauce
>
> 1 tablespoon (16 grams) Worcestershire sauce
>
> Guar or xanthan
>
> 6 tablespoons (60 g) shredded queso quesadilla* or Monterey Jack cheese
>    (optional)

Place the turkey in your slow cooker. (If you can fit more, feel free. My 3-quart slow cooker will only hold 3.)

In a blender, combine the cumin, chili powder, sage, garlic, red pepper flakes, turmeric, chiles, tomato sauce, and Worcestershire sauce. Run it for a minute, then pour the mixture over the turkey. Cover the slow cooker, set it to low, and let it cook for 5 to 6 hours.

When the time's up, remove each turkey leg to a serving plate, thicken the sauce with guar or xanthan, and spoon the sauce over the turkey legs. If you like, sprinkle 2 tablespoons of shredded cheese over each turkey leg and let it melt for a minute or two before serving.

* This is a mild, white Mexican cheese.

**YIELD:** 3 servings, each with: 451 calories, 22 g fat, 54 g protein, 9 g carbohydrate, 2 g dietary fiber, 7 g usable carbs. (Analysis depends on the size of the turkey leg.)

# Turkey with Mushroom Sauce

3 pounds (1.5 kilograms) boneless, skinless turkey breast (in one big hunk, not thin cutlets)

2 tablespoons (28 grams) butter

1/4 cup (16 grams) chopped fresh parsley

2 teaspoons dried tarragon

1/2 teaspoon salt or Vege-Sal

1/4 teaspoon pepper

1 cup (100 grams) sliced mushrooms

1/2 cup (120 milliliters) dry white wine

1 teaspoon chicken bouillon concentrate

Guar or xanthan (optional)

In a big, heavy skillet, sauté the turkey in the butter until it's golden all over. Transfer the turkey to your slow cooker.

Sprinkle the parsley, tarragon, salt or Vege-Sal, and pepper over the turkey. Place the mushrooms on top.

In a bowl, mix the wine and bouillon together until the bouillon dissolves. Pour it over the turkey. Cover the slow cooker, set it to low, and let it cook for 7 to 8 hours.

When the time's up, remove the turkey and put it on a platter. Transfer about half of the mushrooms to a blender and add the liquid from the slow cooker. Blend until the mushrooms are pureed. Scoop the rest of the mushrooms into the dish you plan to use to serve the sauce, add the liquid, and thicken further with guar or xanthan, if needed.

**YIELD:** 8 servings, each with: 281 calories, 14 g fat, 34 g protein, 1 g carbohydrate, trace dietary fiber, 1 g usable carbs.

# CHAPTER FOUR

# Slow Cooker Beef

Tired of steaks and burgers? Use your slow cooker, and you'll be on your way to beef stews, pot roasts, chili, and other classic comfort foods—all waiting when you get home!

# New England Boiled Dinner

This is our traditional St. Patrick's Day dinner, but it's a simple, satisfying one-pot meal on any chilly night. This is easy, but it takes a long time to cook. Do yourself a favor, and assemble it ahead of time. If you have carb-eaters in the family, you can add a few little red boiling potatoes, still in their jackets, to this.

6 small turnips, peeled and quartered

2 large stalks celery, cut into chunks

2 medium onions, cut into chunks

3 pounds (1.5 kilograms) corned beef

1/2 head cabbage, cut into wedges

Spicy brown mustard

Horseradish

Butter

Place the turnips in your slow cooker, along with the celery and the onions. Set the corned beef on top and add water to cover. There will be a seasoning packet with the corned beef—empty it into the slow cooker. Cover the slow cooker, set it to low, and let it cook for 10 to 12 hours. (You can cut the cooking time down to 6 to 8 hours if you set the slow cooker to high, but the low setting yields the most tender results.)

When the time's up, remove the corned beef from the slow cooker with a fork or tongs, put the lid back on the slow cooker to retain heat, put the beef on a platter, and keep it someplace warm. Place the cabbage in the slow cooker with the other vegetables. Re-cover the slow cooker, set it to high, and let it cook for 1/2 hour.

With a slotted spoon, remove all the vegetables and pile them around the corned beef on the platter. Serve with the mustard and horseradish as condiments for the beef and butter for the vegetables.

**YIELD:** 8 servings, each with: 372 calories, 25 g fat, 26 g protein, 9 g carbohydrate, 2 g dietary fiber, 7 g usable carbs.

# Maple-Glazed Corned Beef with Vegetables

This is a trifle less traditional than, but just as good as, the New England Boiled Dinner (see recipe on previous page). The pancake syrup and mustard, plus last-minute glazing under the broiler, give it a new aspect.

6 medium turnips, cut into chunks

2 medium carrots, cut into chunks

1 medium onion, quartered

5 pounds (2.5 kilograms) corned beef brisket

2 cups (470 milliliters) water

1 medium head cabbage, cut into wedges

3 tablespoons (30 grams) sugar-free pancake syrup

1 tablespoon (15 grams) brown mustard

Horseradish

Place the turnips, carrots, and onion in your slow cooker. Place the corned beef on top. Scatter the contents of the accompanying seasoning packet over everything and pour the water over the whole thing. Cover the slow cooker, set it to low, and let it cook for 9 to 10 hours, and a bit more won't hurt!

When the time's up, carefully remove the corned beef and put it on your broiler rack, fatty side up. Use a slotted spoon to skim out the vegetables, put them on a platter, cover, and keep in a warm place.

Place the cabbage in the slow cooker, set it to high, and let it cook for 15 to 20 minutes, or until just tender. (Or you can pour the liquid from the pot into a saucepan and cook the cabbage in it on your stovetop, which is faster.)

While the cabbage is cooking, mix together the pancake syrup and the mustard. Spread the mixture over the corned beef, just the side that is up. When the cabbage is almost done, run the corned beef under your broiler for 2 to 3 minutes, until glazed.

Transfer the cabbage to the platter with a slotted spoon. Slice the corned beef across the grain and serve immediately.

Serve this with horseradish and mustard.

**YIELD:** 12 servings, each with: 416 calories, 28 g fat, 29 g protein, 10 g carbohydrate, 3 g dietary fiber, 7 g usable carbs. (This carb count does not include the polyols in the pancake syrup.)

#  Asian Slow Cooker Short Ribs

Look for black bean sauce in Asian markets or in the international aisle of a big grocery store. You'll only use a little at a time, but it keeps a long time in the fridge, and it adds authenticity to Asian dishes.

6 pounds (3 kilograms) beef short ribs

3 tablespoons (45 milliliters) oil

1 stalk celery, chopped

1/4 cup (30 grams) shredded carrot

1/2 cup (50 grams) chopped onion

2 tablespoons (16 grams) grated ginger root

6 teaspoons Chinese black bean sauce

3 teaspoons chili garlic paste

3 cloves garlic, crushed

1/4 cup (60 milliliters) soy sauce

1 cup (235 milliliters) dry red wine

2 cups (475 milliliters) beef broth

1 teaspoon five-spice powder

1 tablespoon (1.5 grams) Splenda

Guar or xanthan

In a big, heavy skillet, brown the ribs all over in the oil. Transfer the ribs to your slow cooker.

Add the celery, carrot, and onion to the skillet and sauté over medium-high heat until they soften and start to brown. Stir in the ginger, black bean sauce, chili garlic paste, and garlic and sauté for another couple of minutes. Now stir in the soy sauce, wine, broth, five-spice powder, and Splenda. Pour the mixture over the ribs. Cover the slow cooker, set it to low, and let it cook for 6 to 7 hours.

When the time's up, transfer the ribs to a platter and scoop the vegetables into a blender with a slotted spoon. Add 2 cups of the liquid and run the blender till the vegetables are pureed. Thicken the sauce to a heavy cream consistency with guar or xanthan and serve the sauce with the ribs.

**YIELD:** 12 servings, each with: 948 calories, 86 g fat, 35 g protein, 3 g carbohydrate, trace dietary fiber, 3 g usable carbs.

# Balsamic Pot Roast

Balsamic vinegar and rosemary give this pot roast an Italian accent.

3 1/2 pounds (1.75 kilograms) beef round, trimmed of fat

2 tablespoons (28 milliliters) olive oil

1 large onion, sliced

2 cloves garlic, crushed

1 cup (235 milliliters) beef broth

1 teaspoon beef bouillon concentrate

1/4 cup (60 milliliters) balsamic vinegar

1/2 teaspoon dried rosemary, ground

1 cup (260 grams) canned diced tomatoes

Guar or xanthan

In a big, heavy skillet, sear the beef in the oil until browned all over. Transfer the beef to your slow cooker. Scatter the onion and garlic around the beef.

In a bowl, stir together the broth, bouillon, vinegar, and rosemary. Pour the mixture over the beef. Pour the tomatoes on top. Season with pepper. Cover the slow cooker, set it to low, and let it cook for 8 hours.

When the time's up, remove the beef with tongs and place it on a serving platter. Scoop the onions out with a slotted spoon and pile them around the roast. Thicken the juice left in the slow cooker with guar or xanthan and serve it with the beef.

YIELD: 8 servings, each with: 451 calories, 29 g fat, 42 g protein, 5 g carbohydrate, trace dietary fiber, 5 g usable carbs.

#  Bavarian Pot Roast

Given the Bavarian theme and all, I'm thinking Fauxtatoes (see recipe page 239) and cooked cabbage are the obvious side dishes with this.

1 large red onion, sliced 1" thick

2 tablespoons (3 grams) Splenda

¼ teaspoon blackstrap molasses

2 tablespoons (28 milliliters) cider vinegar

1 teaspoon salt

1 teaspoon beef bouillon concentrate

2 ½ pounds (1.25 kilograms) beef round, trimmed of fat and cubed

Guar or xanthan (optional)

Place the onion in your slow cooker.

In a bowl, mix together the Splenda, molasses, vinegar, salt, and bouillon. Pour the mixture over the onion. Place the beef on top. Cover the slow cooker, set it to low, and let it cook for 7 to 8 hours.

When the time's up, thicken the broth with guar or xanthan if desired.

**YIELD:** 8 servings, each with: 297 calories, 18 g fat, 29 g protein, 2 g carbohydrate, trace dietary fiber, 2 g usable carbs.

# Beef and Broccoli

This doesn't come out exactly like stir-fry, but it's still Chinese-y-good, and it's a lot less last-minute trouble.

 1 pound (455 grams) beef round, cut into 1" cubes
 4 ounces (115 grams) canned, sliced mushrooms, drained
 1 medium onion, cut into wedges
 1/2 cup (120 milliliters) beef broth
 1 teaspoon beef bouillon concentrate
 1 tablespoon (1.5 grams) Splenda
 1 teaspoon grated ginger root
 1 tablespoon (14 milliliters) dry sherry
 2 tablespoons (28 milliliters) soy sauce
 1 clove garlic, crushed
 1 teaspoon dark sesame oil
 1 tablespoon (7 grams) sesame seeds
 2 cups (500 grams) frozen broccoli florets
 Guar or xanthan

Combine the beef, mushrooms, onion, broth, bouillon, Splenda, ginger, sherry, soy sauce, garlic, and sesame oil in your slow cooker. Sprinkle the sesame seeds on top. Cover the slow cooker, set it to low, and let it cook for 8 to 10 hours.

When the time's up, add the broccoli to the slow cooker, re-cover the slow cooker, and let it cook for another 30 minutes. Thicken the juices a little with guar or xanthan.

Serve over Cauli-Rice (see recipe page 239) if desired.

**YIELD:** 4 servings, each with: 314 calories, 17 g fat, 29 g protein, 10 g carbohydrate, 4 g dietary fiber, 6 g usable carbs.

#  Beef Carbonnade

Très French!

2 pounds (1 kilogram) beef round, cut into 1" cubes

2 tablespoons (28 milliliters) olive oil

1 large onion, sliced

2 medium carrots, cut 1" thick

2 turnips, cubed

12 ounces (355 milliliters) light beer

1/4 cup (60 milliliters) red wine vinegar

3 tablespoons (4.5 grams) Splenda

1/4 teaspoon blackstrap molasses

1 cup (235 milliliters) beef broth

2 teaspoons beef bouillon concentrate

3 cloves garlic, crushed

2 teaspoons dried thyme

2 teaspoons Worcestershire sauce

1/2 teaspoon pepper

2 bay leaves

Guar or xanthan

In a big, heavy skillet, sear the beef all over in the oil. Place the beef in your slow cooker. Add the onion, carrots, and turnips and stir everything around a bit.

In a bowl, mix together the beer, vinegar, Splenda, molasses, broth, bouillon, garlic, thyme, Worcestershire sauce, and pepper. Pour the mixture into the slow cooker. Throw the bay leaves on top. Cover the slow cooker, set it to low, and let it cook for 8 hours.

When the time's up, remove the bay leaves and add guar or xanthan to thicken the sauce a bit.

You can serve this as is, or, to be more traditional, serve it over Fauxtatoes (see recipe page 239).

**YIELD:** 6 servings, each with: 411 calories, 24 g fat, 34 g protein, 10 g carbohydrate, 2 g dietary fiber, 8 g usable carbs.

# Sauerbrauten

This classic German pot roast takes advance planning, but it's not a lot of work, and it yields impressive results. Don't forget the Fauxtatoes (see recipe page 239) for that gravy!

4 pounds (2 kilograms) boneless beef round or chuck

1 cup (235 milliliters) cider vinegar

1 cup water

1/2 onion, sliced

2 bay leaves

1 teaspoon pepper

1/4 cup (6 grams) Splenda

2 tablespoons (28 milliliters) bacon grease or oil

1/4 teaspoon ground ginger

1 cup (240 grams) light sour cream
  (Use full-fat sour cream if you prefer, but it's no lower carb.)

Guar or xanthan (optional)

Pierce the beef all over with a fork. In a deep, non-reactive bowl (stainless steel, glass, or enamel), combine the vinegar, water, onion, bay leaves, pepper, and Splenda. Place the beef in the marinade and put the bowl in the refrigerator. Marinate the beef for at least 3 days, and 5 or 6 days won't hurt. Turn it over at least once a day, so both sides marinate evenly.

When the time comes to cook your Sauerbrauten, remove the beef from the marinade and pat it dry with paper towels. Reserve the marinade.

In a big, heavy skillet, heat the bacon grease or oil and sear the beef all over. Transfer the beef to your slow cooker.

Scoop the onion and bay leaves out of the marinade with a slotted spoon and put them on top of the beef. Remove 1 cup (235 milliliters) of the marinade from the bowl and add the ginger to it. Pour this over the beef and discard the remaining marinade. Cover the slow cooker, set it to low, and let it cook for 7 to 8 hours.

When the time's up, remove the beef to a serving plate. Stir the sour cream into the liquid in the slow cooker and thicken it if you think it needs it with guar or xanthan. Add salt and pepper to taste and serve the sauce with the beef.

**YIELD:** 10 servings, each with: 407 calories, 26 g fat, 38 g protein, 3 g carbohydrate, trace dietary fiber, 3 g usable carbs.

# Beef Stroganoff

This creamy gravy is fabulous!

2 pounds (1 kilogram) beef round, cut into 1" cubes

1 large onion, chopped

8 ounces (225 grams), canned, sliced mushrooms, undrained

14 ounces (425 milliliters) canned beef broth

1 teaspoon beef bouillon concentrate

2 teaspoons Worcestershire sauce

1 teaspoon paprika

8 ounces (225 grams) cream cheese (regular or light)

8 ounces (225 grams) sour cream (regular or light)

Put the beef in your slow cooker. Put the onion on top, then dump in the mushrooms, liquid and all.

In a bowl, mix the beef broth with the bouillon, Worcestershire sauce, and paprika. Pour the mixture into the slow cooker. Cover the slow cooker, set it to low, and let it cook for 8 to 10 hours.

When the time's up, cut the cream cheese into cubes and stir it into the mixture in the slow cooker until melted. Stir in the sour cream.

Serve over Fauxtatoes (see recipe page 239) or Cauli-Rice (see recipe page 239), if desired. Actually, because noodles are traditional with Stroganoff this would be a good place to serve low-carb pasta, if you have a brand you like.

**NOTE:** This can be made with plain yogurt in place of both the cream cheese and sour cream. After getting everything together in the slow cooker and starting the cooking, place a strainer in a bowl. Line the strainer with a clean coffee filter and pour two 8-ounce containers of plain yogurt into it. Set the strainer and bowl in the refrigerator and let the yogurt drain all day. Whisk the resulting yogurt cheese into your Stroganoff in place of cream cheese and sour cream.

**YIELD:** 8 servings, each with: 413 calories, 31 g fat, 28 g protein, 5 g carbohydrate, 1 g dietary fiber, 4 g usable carbs.

# Beef with Asian Mushroom Sauce

Once you have the Hoisin Sauce on hand, this is very quick to put together. The Hoisin Sauce is a snap, and it keeps well in the fridge.

> 4 ounces (115 grams) sliced mushrooms
> 4 pounds (2 kilograms) beef tip roast
> 1/4 cup (60 milliliters) Hoisin Sauce (see recipe page 233)
> 2 cloves garlic, minced
> 1/2 teaspoon salt
> 1/4 cup (60 milliliters) beef broth
> Guar or xanthan
> 6 tablespoons (35 grams) sliced scallions

Put the mushrooms in your slow cooker and place the beef on top. Spread the Hoisin Sauce over the beef, scatter the garlic and salt over it, and pour in the broth around it. Cover the slow cooker, set it to low, and let it cook for 9 hours.

When the time's up, remove the beef from the slow cooker and put it on a platter. Add guar or xanthan to thicken up the sauce a bit and then pour the sauce into a sauce boat. Slice the beef and serve it with the sauce, topped with the scallions.

**YIELD:** 6 servings, each with: 658 calories, 43 g fat, 61 g protein, 4 g carbohydrate, 1 g dietary fiber, 3 g usable carbs.

#  Short Ribs with Wine and Mushrooms

Short ribs are very flavorful, and this is a simple way to make the most of them.

4 pounds (2 kilograms) beef short ribs

2 bay leaves

1 tablespoon (16 grams) Worcestershire sauce

1 tablespoon (14 milliliters) beef bouillon concentrate

1/2 cup (120 milliliters) dry red wine

8 ounces ( 225 grams) canned mushrooms, drained

Guar or xanthan

Place the ribs in your slow cooker. Add the bay leaves, Worcestershire sauce, and bouillon. Pour the wine over everything. Place the mushrooms on top. Cover the slow cooker, set it to low, and let it cook for 8 to 10 hours.

When the time's up, use a slotted spoon to scoop out the ribs and mushrooms and put them on a platter. There may be a fair amount of grease on the liquid in the pot; it's best to skim it off. Thicken the sauce to taste with guar or xanthan.

Fauxtatoes (see recipe page 239) are the ideal side with this, so you have something to eat all that gravy on!

**YIELD:** 10 servings, each with: 388 calories, 22 g fat, 42 g protein, 1 g carbohydrate, trace dietary fiber, 1 g usable carbs.

# Short Rib Stew

3 pounds (1.5 kilograms) beef short ribs

2 tablespoons (28 milliliters) olive oil

1 medium onion, chopped

8 ounces (225 grams) sliced mushrooms

1 1/2 cups (355 milliliters) beef broth

1/2 teaspoon pepper

1/2 teaspoon dried marjoram

1/2 teaspoon caraway seeds

1 tablespoon (14 milliliters) lemon juice

2 tablespoons (28 milliliters) red wine vinegar

1 teaspoon beef bouillon concentrate

In a big, heavy skillet, brown the ribs all over in the oil over medium-high heat. Transfer the ribs to your slow cooker. In the skillet, over medium-low heat, sauté the onion and mushrooms until they're just softened. Transfer them to the slow cooker, too.

In a bowl, mix together the broth, pepper, marjoram, caraway seeds, lemon juice, vinegar, and bouillon. Pour the mixture over the ribs. Cover the slow cooker, set it to low, and let it cook for 7 to 8 hours.

You can thicken the pot liquid if you like, but I rather like this as is, especially with Fauxtatoes (see recipe page 239).

**YIELD:** 6 servings, each with: 955 calories, 87 g fat, 36 g protein, 5 g carbohydrate, 1 g dietary fiber, 4 g usable carbs.

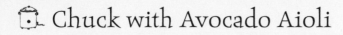# Chuck with Avocado Aioli

This was a big hit with our tester's family!

3 pounds (1.5 kilograms) boneless beef chuck roast

1 tablespoon (14 milliliters) olive oil

1 medium onion, finely chopped

1/2 cup (120 milliliters) water

1 teaspoon beef bouillon concentrate

3 tablespoons (50 grams) Worcestershire sauce

1 teaspoon dried oregano

1 clove garlic, crushed

Avocado Aioli (see recipe on next page)

Season the beef with salt and pepper.

In a big, heavy skillet, sear the beef all over in the oil. Transfer the beef to your slow cooker. Add the onion.

In a bowl, combine the water and bouillon. Pour it over the beef. Add the Worcestershire sauce, oregano, and garlic. Cover the slow cooker, set it to low, and let it cook for 8 hours.

Serve with the Avocado Aioli.

**YIELD:** 8 servings, each with: 381 calories, 28 g fat, 27 g protein, 3 g carbohydrate, trace dietary fiber, 3 g usable carbs.

# Avocado Aioli

You don't have to reserve this for use with the Chuck with Avocado Avioli (see recipe on previous page). Serve it as a dip with vegetables, too. California avocados are the little, black, rough-skinned ones, and they're lower in carbs than the big, green, smooth-skinned Florida avocados.

> 2 ripe California avocados
> 1/4 cup (60 grams) mayonnaise
> 1 tablespoon (14 milliliters) lime juice
> 1-2 cloves garlic, crushed
> 1/4 teaspoon salt

Scoop the avocado flesh into a blender or food processor. Add the mayonnaise, lime juice, garlic, and salt and process until smooth.

**YIELD:** 8 servings, each with: 127 calories, 13 g fat, 1 g protein, 3 g carbohydrate, 2 g dietary fiber, 1 g usable carbs.

# Cube Steaks in Gravy

This is a great down-home, stick-to-the-ribs type of dish.

1 tablespoon (14 milliliters) olive oil

1 1/2 pounds (700 grams) cube steaks

1 medium onion, sliced

8 ounces (225 grams) sliced mushrooms

3 cups (705 milliliters) beef broth

1 tablespoon (14 milliliters) beef bouillon concentrate

Guar or xanthan

In a big, heavy skillet, heat the oil and brown the steaks on both sides.

Put the onion and mushrooms in your slow cooker.

In a bowl, stir the broth and bouillon and pour the mixture over the veggies. Place the steaks on top. Cover the slow cooker, set it to low, and let it cook for 6 to 7 hours.

When the time's up, remove the steaks and thicken the sauce with guar or xanthan to your liking.

Serve with Fauxtatoes (see recipe page 239).

**YIELD:** 6 servings, each with: 297 calories, 17 g fat, 29 g protein, 5 g carbohydrate, 1 g dietary fiber, 4 g usable carbs.

# Easy Italian Beef

This is way easy but full of flavor!

    2 tablespoons (28 milliliters) olive oil
    2 pounds (1 kilogram) beef chuck, trimmed of fat
    1/2 cup (120 milliliters) beef broth
    1 tablespoon (14 milliliters) beef bouillon concentrate
    1 package (.7 ounces/19 grams) Italian salad dressing mix

In a big, heavy skillet, heat the oil over medium-high heat and brown the beef on both sides. Transfer the beef to your slow cooker.

In a bowl, combine the broth, bouillon, and salad dressing mix. Pour the mixture over the beef. Cover the slow cooker, set it to low, and let it cook for 6 to 8 hours.

**YIELD:** 4 servings, each with: 543 calories, 42 g fat, 37 g protein, 1 g carbohydrate, 0 g dietary fiber, 1 g usable carbs.

# Roman Stew

Instead of using the usual Italian seasonings, this was adapted from a historic Roman stew recipe, using spices from the Far East. It's unusual and wonderful.

3 pounds (1.5 kilograms) beef stew meat, cut into 1" cubes

3 tablespoons (45 milliliters) olive oil

4 cloves garlic

2 cups (240 grams) sliced celery

1 teaspoon salt or Vege-Sal

1/4 teaspoon ground cinnamon

1/4 teaspoon ground cloves

1/4 teaspoon pepper

1/8 teaspoon ground allspice

1/8 teaspoon ground nutmeg

14 1/2 ounces (411 grams) canned diced tomatoes, undrained

1/2 cup (120 milliliters) dry red wine

Guar or xanthan (optional)

In a big, heavy skillet, brown the beef in the oil over medium-high heat, in a few batches. Transfer the beef to your slow cooker. Add the garlic and celery to the slow cooker, then sprinkle the salt or Vege-Sal, cinnamon, cloves, pepper, allspice, and nutmeg over the beef and vegetables. Pour the tomatoes and the wine over the beef and vegetables. Cover the slow cooker, set it to low, and let it cook for 7 to 8 hours.

You can thicken the pot juices a little if you like with guar or xanthan, but it's not really necessary.

**YIELD:** 8 servings, each with: 369 calories, 17 g fat, 44 g protein, 5 g carbohydrate, 1 g dietary fiber, 4 g usable carbs.

# Mexican Stew

This Tex-Mex dinner is a simple family-pleaser.

> 2 pounds (1 kilogram) beef stew meat, cut into 1" cubes
> 14 1/2 ounces (411 grams) canned tomatoes with green chiles
> 1/2 cup (50 grams) sliced onion
> 1 teaspoon chili powder
> 1 envelope (1 1/4 ounces/35 grams) taco seasoning mix
> 15 ounces (425 grams) canned black soybeans
> 1/2 cup (115 grams) sour cream

Put the beef, tomatoes, onion, and chili powder in your slow cooker. Cover the slow cooker, set it to low, and let it cook for 8 to 9 hours.

Stir in the taco seasoning and soybeans. Re-cover the slow cooker, turn it to high, and let it cook for another 20 minutes. Place a dollop of sour cream on each serving.

This makes 6 generous servings, and it could even serve 8.

**YIELD:** 6 servings, each with: 399 calories, 18 g fat, 46 g protein, 12 g carbohydrate, 5 g dietary fiber, 7 g usable carbs.

#  Comfort Food Casserole

This is one of those meal-in-a-bowl sorts of things that just seem—well, comforting, somehow. I've found that slow cooking really brings out the best in turnips. They end up remarkably like potatoes.

1 1/2 pounds (700 grams) ground round

1 tablespoon (14 milliliters) oil

1 medium onion, chopped

4 cloves garlic, crushed

4 stalks celery, diced

1 cup (235 milliliters) beef broth

1 teaspoon beef bouillon concentrate

1/2 teaspoon salt or Vege-Sal

1 teaspoon pepper

2 teaspoons dried oregano

1 teaspoon dry mustard

2 tablespoons (32 grams) tomato paste

4 ounces (115 grams) cream cheese

3 turnips, cubed

3/4 cup (85 grams) shredded cheddar cheese

In a big, heavy skillet, brown and crumble the beef over medium-high heat. Pour off the fat and transfer the beef to your slow cooker.

Add the oil to the skillet and reduce the heat to medium-low. Add the onion, garlic, and celery and sauté until they're just softened. Add the broth, bouillon, salt or Vege-Sal, pepper, oregano, dry mustard, and tomato paste and stir. Now add the cream cheese, using the edge of a spatula to cut the cream cheese into chunks. Let this mixture simmer, stirring occasionally, until the cream cheese is melted.

Meanwhile add the turnips to the slow cooker.

When the cream cheese has melted into the sauce, pour the sauce into the slow cooker. Stir until the ground beef and turnips are coated. Cover the slow cooker, set it to low, and let it cook for 6 hours. Serve with cheddar cheese on top.

**YIELD:** 6 servings, each with: 549 calories, 40 g fat, 35 g protein, 12 g carbohydrate, 3 g dietary fiber, 9 g usable carbs.

# Firehouse Chili

Here's a crowd-pleaser! I served this on a rainy afternoon at our local camp-ground and made a lot of friends! You could halve this, but you'd be left with a half a can of soybeans, and you know you'll eat it up, so why bother?

2 pounds (1 kilogram) ground chuck

1 1/2 cups (150 grams) chopped onion

4 cloves garlic, crushed

3 tablespoons (21 grams) chili powder

3 teaspoons paprika

4 teaspoons ground cumin

1/4 cup (60 grams) Dana's No-Sugar Ketchup (see recipe page 228)
   or purchased low-carb ketchup

2 tablespoons (32 grams) tomato paste

14 1/2 ounces (411 grams) canned diced tomatoes

12 ounces (355 milliliters) light beer

1 teaspoon Splenda

2 1/2 teaspoons salt

15 ounces (425 grams) canned black soybeans

In a big, heavy skillet, brown and crumble the beef over medium-high heat. Drain it and place it in your slow cooker. Add the onion, garlic, chili powder, paprika, cumin, ketchup, tomato paste, tomatoes, beer, Splenda, salt, and soybeans. Stir everything up. Cover the slow cooker, set it to low, and let it cook for 8 hours.

This is good with shredded cheese and sour cream. What chili isn't? But it also stands on its own very well.

YIELD: 10 servings, each with: 329 calories, 21 g fat, 21 g protein, 12 g carbohydrate, 4 g dietary fiber, 8 g usable carbs.

# Carne all'Ungherese

The original recipe, from which I adapted this, said it was an Italian version of a Hungarian stew. Whatever it is, it's good!

1/4 cup (60 milliliters) olive oil

1 1/2 pounds (700 grams) beef stew meat, cut into 1" cubes

1 medium onion, chopped

1 green pepper, cut into strips

2 cloves garlic, crushed

1 cup (235 milliliters) beef broth

1 teaspoon beef bouillon concentrate

1 teaspoon dried marjoram

1 tablespoon (16 grams) tomato paste

1 tablespoon (7 grams) paprika

1 tablespoon (28 milliliters) lemon juice

1/2 cup (125 grams) plain yogurt

In a big, heavy skillet, heat a tablespoon or two of the oil over medium-high heat. Start browning the stew meat. It will take two or three batches; add more oil as you need it. Transfer each batch of browned meat to your slow cooker as it's done.

When all the meat is browned, put the last of the oil in the skillet, reduce the heat to medium-low, and add the onion. Sauté the onion until it's just softening and add it to the slow cooker. Add the green pepper to the slow cooker.

In a bowl, mix together the garlic, broth, bouillon, marjoram, tomato paste, paprika, and lemon juice, stirring until the bouillon and tomato paste are dissolved. Pour the mixture over the meat and onions. Cover the slow cooker, set it to low, and let it cook for 6 to 7 hours.

When the time's up, stir in the yogurt.

Serve over Fauxtatoes (see recipe page 239).

**YIELD:** 5 servings, each with: 382 calories, 22 g fat, 38 g protein, 7 g carbohydrate, 1 g dietary fiber, 6 g usable carbs. (Analysis does not include Fauxtatoes.)

# ☐ Swiss Steak

Here's a no-work version of this old-time favorite.

> 1 large onion, sliced
>
> 3 pounds (1.5 kilograms) beef round
>
> 1 tablespoon (14 milliliters) beef bouillon concentrate
>
> 8 ounces (235 milliliters) vegetable juice (such as V8)
>
> 2 stalks celery, sliced
>
> Guar or xanthan (optional)

Place the onion in your slow cooker. Place the beef on top.

In a bowl, stir the bouillon into the vegetable juice. Pour the mixture over the beef. Scatter the celery on top. Cover the slow cooker, set it to low, and let it cook for 8 to 10 hours.

When the time's up, thicken the juices with guar or xanthan if desired.

Serve over pureed cauliflower.

**YIELD:** 8 servings, each with: 360 calories, 22 g fat, 35 g protein, 3 g carbohydrate, 1 g dietary fiber, 2 g usable carbs.

#  Beef and Zucchini Stew

Don't try adding the zukes at the beginning, or they'll cook to a mush! Put out some vegetables and dip for the ravening hoards, and sip a glass of wine while you're waiting that last hour.

2 pounds (1 kilogram) boneless beef chuck, trimmed of fat and cubed

1 medium onion, sliced

1 large red bell pepper, cut into 1" squares

1 large green bell pepper, cut into 1" squares

1 cup (250 grams) no-sugar-added spaghetti sauce (I suggest Hunt's.)

1/2 cup (120 milliliters) beef broth

1/2 teaspoon beef bouillon concentrate

1 1/2 pounds (700 grams) zucchini, cut into 1/2" slices

Guar or xanthan (optional)

In your slow cooker, combine the beef with the onion and peppers.

In a bowl, stir together the spaghetti sauce, broth, and bouillon. Pour the mixture over the beef and vegetables and stir. Cover the slow cooker, set it to low, and let it cook for 9 hours.

Turn the slow cooker to high, stir in the zucchini, re-cover, and let it cook for 1 more hour.

When the time's up, thicken the sauce with guar or xanthan if needed.

**YIELD:** 6 servings, each with: 367 calories, 24 g fat, 27 g protein, 10 g carbohydrate, 3 g dietary fiber, 7 g usable carbs.

# Chipotle Brisket

Our tester, who loved this recipe, halved it. You can feel free to do the same.

> 4 pounds (2 kilograms) beef brisket, cut into pieces if necessary
>   to fit into your slow cooker
> 2 tablespoons (28 milliliters) olive oil
> 1 medium onion, thinly sliced
> 4 stalks celery, thinly sliced
> 4 cloves garlic, crushed
> 1 tablespoon (11 grams) dry mustard
> 1 tablespoon (4 grams) dried oregano
> 1 teaspoon ground cumin
> 2 teaspoons pepper
> 1 teaspoon salt or Vege-Sal
> 16 ounces (455 grams) canned tomato sauce
> 1/2 cup (120 milliliters) beef broth
> 1 teaspoon beef bouillon concentrate
> 1/4 cup (60 milliliters) red wine vinegar
> 1/2 cup (12 grams) Splenda
> 1/2 teaspoon blackstrap molasses
> 2 chipotle chiles canned in adobo sauce
> 2 bay leaves
> Guar or xanthan

In a big, heavy skillet, brown the beef all over in the oil over medium-high heat. Transfer the beef to your slow cooker.

Add the onion and celery to the skillet and sauté until softened. Stir in the garlic, dry mustard, oregano, cumin, pepper, and salt or Vege-Sal and sauté for another minute or two. Transfer the mixture to the slow cooker, on top of the brisket.

In a blender or food processor, combine the tomato sauce, broth, bouillon, vinegar, Splenda, molasses, and chipotles and blend until smooth.

Put the bay leaves in the slow cooker, on top of the beef, and pour the sauce over the whole thing. Cover the slow cooker, set it to low, and let it cook for 12 hours.

When the time's up, remove the beef to a platter. Thicken the sauce to taste with guar or xanthan and serve the sauce over the beef.

**YIELD:** 8 servings, each with: 779 calories, 64 g fat, 41 g protein, 8 g carbohydrate, 2 g dietary fiber, 6 g usable carbs.

# Simple Salsa Beef

Here's one of those super-simple dump-and-go recipes. It's great for a day when you didn't get dinner in the slow cooker the night before!

3 turnips, peeled and cubed

1 pound (455 grams) baby carrots

3 pounds (1.5 kilograms) beef arm pot roast

2 cups (520 grams) salsa

Guar or xanthan (optional)

Put the turnips and carrots in your slow cooker, then place the beef on top. Pour the salsa over the lot. Cover the slow cooker, set it to low, and let it cook for 8 to 10 hours.

When the time's up, remove the beef and pull it apart into shreds with two forks. Scoop the vegetables out onto serving plates with a slotted spoon. Pile the beef on top. If desired, thicken the sauce with a little guar or xanthan. Spoon the sauce over the vegetables and beef.

**YIELD:** 8 servings, each with: 200 calories, 5 g fat, 26 g protein, 11 g carbohydrate, 3 g dietary fiber, 8 g usable carbs.

# Oxtails Pontchartrain

This has a lot of New Orleans elements, including some serious heat, so I named it after Lake Pontchartrain. Oxtails are bony, but very flavorful, and they take very well to the slow cooker. If you haven't had oxtails, don't fear them; they're just muscle meat, like a steak or a roast. It's just that there's a high bone-to-meat ratio.

> 4 pounds (2 kilograms) beef oxtails
>
> 3 tablespoons (18 grams) Cajun seasoning
>
> 2 tablespoons (28 milliliters) olive oil
>
> 3 large banana peppers, sliced
>
> 1 medium onion, sliced
>
> 1 medium carrot, shredded
>
> 2 stalks celery, sliced
>
> 1 clove garlic, crushed
>
> 1 cup (235 milliliters) dry red wine
>
> 1/4 cup (60 milliliters) brandy
>
> 1 1/2 teaspoons dried thyme
>
> 3 bay leaves
>
> 14 1/2 ounces (411 grams) canned diced tomatoes
>
> 2 chipotle chiles canned in adobo sauce, chopped
> (You can use just one if you'd like to cut the heat a bit.)

Sprinkle the oxtails all over with the Cajun seasoning.

In a big, heavy skillet, heat the oil and brown the oxtails all over. Transfer the oxtails to your slow cooker.

Add the peppers, onion, carrot, celery, and garlic to the skillet and sauté them until they're just softened. Add them to the slow cooker, too, and mix them in with the oxtails.

Pour the wine and brandy in the skillet and stir it around. Stir in the thyme and add the bay leaves, tomatoes, and chipotles. Stir this all up and pour it over the oxtails and veggies. Cover the slow cooker, set it to low, and let it cook for 8 hours.

**YIELD:** 6 servings each with: 935 calories, 48 g fat, 96 g protein, 13 g carbohydrate, 3 g dietary fiber, 10 g usable carbs.

#  3-Minute Slow Cooker Pot Roast

This recipe, originally from *15-Minute Low-Carb Recipes*, is very 1965, but it's still incredibly easy, and it tastes great.

> 8 ounces (225 grams) sliced mushrooms
> 2–3 pounds (1–1.5 kilograms) boneless chuck pot roast
> 1 envelope (1 ounce/23 grams) French onion soup mix
> 1/2 cup (120 milliliters) dry red wine
> Guar or xanthan

Place the mushrooms in the bottom of your slow cooker and add the beef on top of them.

In a bowl, mix together the onion soup mix and wine and pour it into the slow cooker. Cover the slow cooker, set it to low, and let it cook for 8 hours.

When the time's up, remove the beef (carefully—it will be very tender) and use the guar or xanthan to thicken the juices in the slow cooker. Serve this gravy with the pot roast.

**YIELD:** 6 servings, each with: 358 calories, 24 g fat, 25 g protein, 6 g carbohydrate, 1 g dietary fiber, 5 g usable carbs. (This analysis assumes you use a 2-pound roast and that you eat every drop of the gravy.)

# Pepperoncini Beef

Pepperoncini are hot-but-not-scorching pickled Italian salad peppers. You'll find these in the same aisle as the olives and pickles. They make this beef very special.

2–3 pounds (1–1.5 kilograms) boneless chuck pot roast
1 cup (120 grams) pepperoncini peppers, undrained
1/2 medium onion, chopped
Guar or xanthan

Place the beef in your slow cooker, pour the peppers on top, and strew the onion over that. Cover the slow cooker, set it to low, and let it cook for 8 hours.

When the time's up, remove the beef, put it on a platter, and use a slotted spoon to scoop out the peppers and pile them on top of the beef. Thicken the juices in the pot with the guar or xanthan. Add salt and pepper to taste and serve the sauce with the beef.

**YIELD:** 6 servings, each with: 325 calories, 24 g fat, 24 g protein, 3 g carbohydrate, trace dietary fiber, 3 g usable carbs. (This analysis is for a 2-pound roast.)

# Beef in Beer

Here's a simple recipe from *500 Low-Carb Recipes*. The tea, the beer, and the long, slow cooking make this as tender as can be. I've changed this just a little. Originally, you dredged the beef in soy powder or low-carb bake mix, but I've decided that's inessential. And it's another step, and a messy one at that.

> 2-3 tablespoons (28-42 milliliters) olive oil
>
> 2 pounds (905 grams) boneless beef round roast
>
> 1 medium onion, sliced
>
> 8 ounces (225 grams) canned tomato sauce
>
> 12 ounces (355 milliliters) light beer
>
> 1 teaspoon instant tea powder
>
> 4 ounces (115 grams) canned mushrooms, drained
>
> 2 cloves garlic, crushed

Heat oil in a big, heavy skillet over medium-high heat and sear the beef until it's brown all over. Transfer the beef to your slow cooker.

In the oil left in the skillet, fry the onion for a few minutes and add that to the slow cooker, too.

Pour the tomato sauce and beer over the beef. Sprinkle the tea over it and add the mushrooms and garlic. Cover the slow cooker, set it to low, and let it cook for 8 to 9 hours.

This is good served with Fauxtatoes (recipe page 239).

**YIELD:** 6 servings, each with: 374 calories, 24 g fat, 28 g protein, 7 g carbohydrate, 2 g dietary fiber, 5 g usable carbs.

# Peking Slow Cooker Pot Roast

This sounds nuts, but it tastes great! This recipe, originally from *500 Low-Carb Recipes*, takes starting ahead, but it's not a lot of work.

- 3–5 pounds (1.5–2.5 kilograms) beef roast (round, chuck, or rump)
- 5 or 6 cloves garlic, sliced thin
- 8 ounces (235 milliliters) cider vinegar
- 1 cup (235 milliliters) water
- 1 small onion, thinly sliced
- 1 1/2 cups (355 milliliters) strong coffee (instant works fine)
- 1 teaspoon guar or xanthan

At least 24 to 36 hours before you want to actually cook your roast, stick holes in the beef with a thin-bladed knife and insert a garlic slice into each hole. Put the beef in a big bowl and pour the vinegar and the water over it. Put it in the refrigerator and let it sit there for a day or so, turning it over when you think of it so the whole thing marinates.

On the morning of the day you want to serve your roast, pour off the marinade and put the beef in your slow cooker. Place the onion on top of the beef. Pour the coffee over the beef and onion. Cover the slow cooker, set it to low, and let it cook for 8 hours for a smaller roast or up to 10 hours for a larger one.

When the time's up, remove the beef carefully from the cooker. (It will now be so tender it's likely to fall apart.) Scoop out 2 cups (475 milliliters) of the liquid and some of the onions and put them in a blender with the guar or xanthan. Blend for few seconds, then pour the mixture into a saucepan set over high heat. Boil this sauce hard for about 5 minutes to reduce it a bit. Add salt and pepper to the sauce to taste. (It's amazing the difference the salt and pepper make here; I didn't like the flavor of this sauce until I added the salt and pepper, and then I liked it a lot.) Slice the beef and serve it with this sauce.

**WARNING:** Do not make this with a tender cut of beef! This recipe will tenderize the toughest cut; a tender one will practically dissolve. Use inexpensive, tough cuts, and prepare to be amazed at how fork-tender they get.

**YIELD:** 12 servings, each with: 324 calories, 24 g fat, 24 g protein, 3 g carbohydrate, trace dietary fiber, 3 g usable carbs. (This analysis is for a 4-pound boneless roast.)

# Good Low-Carb Slow Cooked Short Ribs

This was one of the first recipes I adapted from Peg Bracken's *I Hate To Cook Book*, aka The World's Funniest Cookbook (and also one of the most useful.) It was higher carb, and it wasn't originally a slow cooker recipe, but it adapted well to both!

8 ounces (225 grams) canned tomato sauce

3/4 cup (175 milliliters) water

2 tablespoons (28 milliliters) wine or cider vinegar

4 tablespoons (60 milliliters) soy sauce

2 teaspoons Splenda

3–4 pounds (1.5–2 kilograms) beef short ribs

1 large onion, sliced

Guar or xanthan (optional)

In a bowl, mix together the tomato sauce, water, vinegar, soy sauce, and Splenda.

Put the ribs in your slow cooker. Place the onion on top of the ribs. Pour the sauce over the onion and ribs. Cover the slow cooker, set it to low, and let it cook for 8 to 9 hours. (If you put the ribs in thawed, cut about 1 hour off the cooking time.)

When the time's up, thicken the sauce with guar or xanthan if you prefer. (This recipe gives you tremendously tasty ribs in a thin but flavorful sauce—it's more like a broth. You can thicken it a bit with guar or xanthan, but I rather like it as it is.)

**YIELD:** 7 servings, each with: 559 calories, 31 g fat, 61 g protein, 5 g carbohydrate, 1 g dietary fiber, 4 g usable carbs. (This analysis is for 3 pounds of ribs. The total carbs will vary with how much of the sauce you eat, because most of the carbs are in there. Furthermore, that calorie count assumes that you eat all of the fat that cooks off of the ribs—which I wouldn't suggest.)

# CHAPTER FIVE

# Slow Cooker Pork

This is one big chapter, and with good reason. Pork is delicious, nutritious, versatile, and slow cooks really well. You'll find everything from simple family suppers to company food in this chapter!

# Braised Pork with Fennel

This was one of my first great slow-cooking triumphs, and it still ranks as one of the two or three best dishes I've ever cooked in my slow cooker. This is easily good enough to serve to company. By the way, some grocery stores label "fennel" as "anise." It looks like a bulb at the bottom, with celery-like stalks above, and feathery foliage. The stems are tough, but the foliage can be chopped up in salads or used as a garnish. It has a wonderful licorice-like taste.

4 pounds (2 kilograms) pork shoulder roast

2 tablespoons (28 milliliters) olive oil

1 medium onion, sliced

1 bulb fennel, sliced

1 cup (235 milliliters) cider vinegar

3 tablespoons (4.5 grams) Splenda

1 cup (260 grams) canned diced tomatoes, drained

1 cup (235 milliliters) chicken broth

1 teaspoon chicken bouillon concentrate

2 cloves garlic, crushed

1/2 teaspoon dried thyme

1/2 teaspoon red pepper flakes, or to taste

Guar or xanthan

In a big, heavy skillet, sear the pork in the oil over medium-high heat until it's brown all over. (This will take 20 minutes or so.) Transfer the pork to your slow cooker.

Pour off all but about 1 tablespoon of fat from the skillet and reduce the heat to medium-low. Sauté the onion and fennel until they're just getting a little golden. Transfer them to the slow cooker, too.

In a bowl, mix together the vinegar and Splenda. Pour the mixture over the pork. Add the tomatoes.

In a bowl, mix together the broth and bouillon until the bouillon dissolves. Stir in the garlic, thyme, and red pepper. Pour this over the pork, too. Cover the slow cooker, set it to low, and let it cook for 8 hours.

When the time's up, remove the pork from the slow cooker and place it on a serving platter. Using a slotted spoon, scoop out the vegetables and pile them around the pork. Cover the platter with foil and put it in a warm place.

Ladle the liquid from the slow cooker into a saucepan. Place it over the highest heat and boil it hard for 5 to 7 minutes, to reduce the sauce a bit. Add some guar or xanthan to thicken the sauce just a bit. (You want it to be about the texture of half-and-half, not a thick gravy.) Serve the sauce over the pork and vegetables.

**YIELD:** 6 servings, each with: 621 calories, 46 g fat, 41 g protein, 10 g carbohydrate, 2 g dietary fiber, 8 g usable carbs.

# ⬛ Easy Pork Roast

This is basic, which is a strength, not a weakness. It would be a great supper with a big salad.

>   3 pounds (1.5 kilograms) boneless pork loin
>   2 tablespoons (28 milliliters) olive oil
>   8 ounces (225 grams) tomato sauce
>   1/4 cup (60 milliliters) soy sauce
>   1/2 cup (120 milliliters) chicken broth
>   1/2 cup (12 grams) Splenda
>   2 teaspoons dry mustard
>   Guar or xanthan (optional)

In a big, heavy skillet, brown the pork on all sides in the oil. Transfer the pork to your slow cooker.

In a bowl, mix together the tomato sauce, soy sauce, broth, Splenda, and dry mustard. Pour the mixture over the pork. Cover the slow cooker, set it to low, and let it cook for 8 to 9 hours.

When the time's up, remove the pork to a serving platter. Thicken the pot liquid, if needed, with guar or xanthan. Serve the juice with the pork.

**YIELD:** 8 servings, each with: 301 calories, 14 g fat, 37 g protein, 4 g carbohydrate, 1 g dietary fiber, 3 g usable carbs.

# Pork Roast with Apricot Sauce

Here's a fabulous Sunday dinner for the family—with very little work.

2 1/2 pounds (1.25 kilograms) boneless pork loin

2 tablespoons (28 milliliters) olive oil

1/3 cup (35 grams) chopped onion

3/4 cup (175 milliliters) chicken broth

1/4 cup (80 grams) low-sugar apricot preserves

1 tablespoon (14 milliliters) balsamic vinegar

1 tablespoon (14 milliliters) lemon juice

1 tablespoon (1.5 grams) Splenda

Guar or xanthan

In a big, heavy skillet, sear the pork all over in the oil. Transfer the pork to your slow cooker. Scatter the onion around it.

In a bowl, mix together the broth, preserves, vinegar, lemon juice, and Splenda. Pour the mixture over the pork. Cover the slow cooker, set it to low, and let it cook for 7 hours.

When the time's up, remove the pork and put it on a serving platter. Season the juices with salt and pepper to taste. Thicken the juices with guar or xanthan. Ladle the juices into a sauce boat to serve.

**YIELD:** 6 servings, each with: 338 calories, 17 g fat, 40 g protein, 5 g carbohydrate, trace dietary fiber, 5 g usable carbs.

# Pork Roast with Creamy Mushroom Gravy and Vegetables

Here's a great down-home dinner the family will love!

  2 1/2 pounds (1.25 kilograms) boneless pork loin
  1/2 cup (60 grams) sliced carrots
  4 ounces (115 grams) sliced mushrooms
  10 ounces (280 grams) frozen cross-cut green beans, unthawed
  1 tablespoon (14 milliliters) beef bouillon concentrate
  2 tablespoons (28 milliliters) water
  14 1/2 ounces (411 grams) canned tomatoes with roasted garlic
  Guar or xanthan
  1/2 cup (120 milliliters) heavy cream

Put the pork in the bottom of your slow cooker. Surround the pork with the carrots, mushrooms, and green beans. (Don't bother thawing the green beans, just whack the package hard on the counter before opening, so the beans are all separated.)

In a bowl, dissolve the bouillon in the water. Stir in the tomatoes. Pour the mixture over the pork and vegetables. Cover the slow cooker, set it to low, and let it cook for 8 to 9 hours.

When the time's up, remove the pork and vegetables to a platter. Thicken the juices in the pot with guar or xanthan, then whisk in the cream. Add salt and pepper to taste. Serve the juices with the pork and vegetables.

**YIELD:** 8 servings, each with: 284 calories, 19 g fat, 23 g protein, 5 g carbohydrate, 1 g dietary fiber, 4 g usable carbs.

#  Orange Rosemary Pork

One day I saw the adorable Rachael Ray (whose Food Network show I love) grilling some pork chops for one of her 30-minute meals, and she was saying that orange and rosemary were great for basting pork. Well, hey, Rachael knows what she's talking about, so I decided to borrow those flavors for a low-carb slow cooker dish. Oh, boy, did it work out well! Thanks for the idea, Rachael!

1 1/2 pounds (700 grams) boneless pork loin

2 tablespoons (28 milliliters) olive oil

1/4 cup (60 milliliters) white wine vinegar

1/4 cup (60 milliliters) lemon juice

3 tablespoons (4.5 grams) Splenda

1/4 teaspoon orange extract

1/2 teaspoon ground, dried rosemary

1 clove garlic, crushed

1 teaspoon soy sauce

1/4 teaspoon pepper

1/4 teaspoon salt or Vege-Sal

In a big, heavy skillet, brown the pork in the oil over medium-high heat. Transfer the pork to your slow cooker.

In a bowl, stir together the vinegar, lemon juice, Splenda, orange extract, rosemary, garlic, soy sauce, pepper, and salt or Vege-Sal and pour over the pork. Cover the slow cooker, set it to low, and let it cook for 5 to 6 hours.

**YIELD:** 4 servings, each with: 317 calories, 23 g fat, 23 g protein, 3 g carbohydrate, trace dietary fiber, 3 g usable carbs.

# Pork with Cabbage

Need I point out that this recipe is for cabbage lovers?

> 4 pounds (2 kilograms) boneless pork shoulder roast, trimmed of fat
>
> 2 tablespoons (28 milliliters) olive oil
>
> 2 carrots, cut into 1" pieces
>
> 2 cloves garlic, crushed
>
> 2 stalks celery, cut 1/2" thick
>
> 1 envelope (1 ounce/23 grams) onion soup mix
>
> 1 1/2 cups (355 milliliters) water
>
> 1 1/2 pounds (700 grams) cabbage, coarsely chopped
>
> Guar or xanthan

In a big, heavy skillet, start browning the pork in the oil.

Place the carrots, garlic, and celery in your slow cooker. Add the soup mix and water.

When the pork is brown all over, put it on top of the vegetables in the slow cooker. Cover the slow cooker, set it to low, and let it cook for 7 hours.

When the time's up, stir in the cabbage, pushing it down into the liquid. Re-cover the slow cooker and let it cook for another 45 minutes to 1 hour

Remove the pork and put it on a platter. Use a slotted spoon to pile the vegetables around the pork. Thicken the liquid in the slow cooker with guar or xanthan. Add salt and pepper to taste. Pour the liquid into a sauce boat and serve with the pork and vegetables.

**YIELD:** 8 servings, each with: 478 calories, 35 g fat, 31 g protein, 10 g carbohydrate, 3 g dietary fiber, 7 g usable carbs.

# Pork with Rutabaga

If you haven't tried rutabaga, you simply must. Also sometimes called a "swede," or a "yellow turnip," rutabaga is similar to a turnip, except that it has an entrancing bitter-sweet flavor. Anyway, it's fun confusing grocery store checkout clerks who can't figure out what that big yellow root is! It's actually delicious to make this with half rutabaga and half a fresh, cubed pumpkin, but it's just not possible to find fresh pumpkin some seasons of the year.

2 1/2 pounds (1.25 kilograms) rutabaga, peeled and cubed

3 pounds (1.5 kilograms) boneless pork shoulder roast, tied or netted

1/2 teaspoon blackstrap molasses

1/2 cup (12 grams) Splenda

1/4 teaspoon cayenne

1 clove garlic, minced

Put the rutabaga in the bottom of your slow cooker. Put the pork on top. Drizzle the molasses over the pork and rutabega.

In a bowl, mix together the Splenda, cayenne, and garlic. Sprinkle the mixture over the pork and rutabaga. Cover the slow cooker, set it to low, and let it cook for 8 to 9 hours.

When the time's up, remove the pork from the slow cooker, cut off the string or net, and slice or pull the pork apart. Serve the pork over the rutabaga with the pot liquid.

YIELD: 6 servings, each with: 472 calories, 31 g fat, 32 g protein, 16 g carbohydrate, 5 g dietary fiber, 11 g usable carbs.

# ⊙ "Honey" Mustard Ham

You may wonder how to roast a ham when you're not going to be around for hours to tend the oven. In your slow cooker, of course. You'll need a big slow cooker for this.

> 5 pounds (2.5 kilograms) fully cooked, bone-in ham
> 1/3 cup (75 milliliters) apple cider vinegar
> 1/2 cup (12 grams) Splenda
> 1 tablespoon (15 grams) brown mustard
> 1/2 teaspoon blackstrap molasses
> 1 teaspoon water

Place the ham in your slow cooker.

In a bowl, mix together the vinegar and 2 tablespoons of the Splenda. Add the mixture to the slow cooker. In the same bowl, mix together the mustard, molasses, remaining Splenda, and water and spread the mixture over the ham. Cover the slow cooker, set it to low, and let it cook for 7 hours.

**YIELD:** 6 servings, each with: 683 calories, 41 g fat, 68 g protein, 6 g carbohydrate, trace dietary fiber, 6 g usable carbs.

# ☺ Ham with Rutabaga and Turnips

If you're roasting a ham in your slow cooker, you may as well roast your vegetables, too, right?

4 turnips, cubed

1 1/2 pounds (700 grams) rutabaga, peeled and cubed

6 1/2 pounds (3.25 kilograms) shank half ham

Put the turnips and rutabaga in the bottom of your slow cooker. Place the ham on top, flat side down. Cover the slow cooker, set it to low, and let it cook for 5 to 6 hours. Again, you'll need a big slow cooker.

**YIELD:** 10 servings, each with: 674 calories, 51 g fat, 43 g protein, 9 g carbohydrate, 3 g dietary fiber, 6 g usable carbs.

# Creamy Ham Casserole

I made this up to use the end of a ham I'd slow cooked, and it was a hit with my husband.

- 1 head cauliflower
- 1 medium onion, chopped
- 1 large stalk celery, with leaves
- 2 cups (475 milliliters) Carb Countdown dairy beverage
- 1 cup (235 milliliters) chicken broth
- 6 teaspoons guar or xanthan
- 1 teaspoon dry mustard
- 1 teaspoon salt or Vege-Sal
- 1/2 teaspoon pepper
- 8 ounces (225 grams) Gruyère cheese, shredded

Run the cauliflower through the slicing blade of your food processor. Transfer it to a bowl and replace the slicing disc with the S-blade. Chop the onion and celery fine in the food processor.

With a hand blender or regular blender, blend the Carb Countdown and broth. Add the guar or xanthan and blend it until there are no lumps. Pour the mixture it into a saucepan and heat it over medium-low heat. (If you do have a hand blender, you may as well just dump the Carb Countdown and the chicken broth in the saucepan and use the hand blender to blend in the thickener in the pot to save a little dishwashing.) Stir in the dry mustard, salt or Vege-Sal, and pepper. When the sauce is hot, stir in the cheese, a little at a time, until it's all melted. Turn off the burner.

Spray your slow cooker with nonstick cooking spray. Put in a layer of cauliflower, a lighter layer of onion and celery, then a generous layer of ham. Repeat these layers until everything's gone and the slow cooker is full. Pour half of the sauce over the top. It won't immediately flow down into the food in the slow cooker, so poke down into it several times with the handle of a rubber scraper or spoon, piercing the layers to the bottom. The sauce will start to seep down. When there's more room on top, pour in the rest of the sauce, and poke down through the layers again. Cover the slow cooker, set it to low, and let it cook for 6 to 7 hours.

**YIELD:** 8 servings, each with: 287 calories, 19 g fat, 24 g protein, 5 g carbohydrate, 1 g dietary fiber, 4 g usable carbs.

#  Sweet and Sour Pork

Here's another stir-fry dish turned into a slow cooker meal. This lacks the chunks of pineapple you often find in sweet-and-sour dishes. They're just too high carb. But the crushed pineapple in the sauce gives the right flavor!

1 1/2 pounds (700 grams) boneless pork loin, cut into 1" cubes

1 green bell pepper, diced

1/4 cup (6 grams) Splenda

1 tablespoon (8 grams) grated ginger root

1 clove garlic, crushed

1/4 cup (60 milliliters) rice vinegar

3 tablespoons (45 milliliters) soy sauce

1/4 teaspoon blackstrap molasses

1/3 cup (65 grams) canned crushed pineapple in juice

1/2 head cauliflower

Guar or xanthan

Put the pork and pepper in your slow cooker.

In a bowl, mix together the Splenda, ginger, garlic, vinegar, soy sauce, molasses, and pineapple. Pour the mixture over the pork and pepper. Cover the slow cooker, set it on low, and let it cook for 6 hours.

When the time's up, run the cauliflower through the shredding blade of a food processor and put it in a microwaveable casserole dish with a lid. Add a couple of tablespoons of water, cover, and microwave on high for 7 minutes. This is your Cauli-Rice!

Meanwhile, thicken up the pot juices with guar or xanthan until they're about the texture of commercial Chinese food. Serve the pork mixture over the Cauli-Rice.

**YIELD:** 4 servings, each with: 283 calories, 11 g fat, 36 g protein, 9 g carbohydrate, 1 g dietary fiber, 8 g usable carbs.

# Curried Pork Stew

This is not terribly authentic, but it's awfully good. Try one of the chutneys (see recipe pages 208 and 210) with this.

> 1 pound (455 grams) boneless pork loin, cubed
> 1/2 teaspoon salt
> 2 tablespoons (12 grams) curry powder
> 1 tablespoon (14 milliliters) olive oil
> 1 onion, sliced
> 2 small turnips, cubed
> 1 cup (260 grams) canned diced tomatoes
> 1/2 cup (120 milliliters) cider vinegar
> 2 tablespoons (3 grams) Splenda
> 2 cups (300 grams) diced cauliflower

Season the pork with the salt and sprinkle with 1 tablespoon of the curry powder.

In a big, heavy skillet, heat the oil and brown the pork over medium-high heat.

Place the onion and turnips in your slow cooker. Top with the pork and tomatoes.

In a bowl, stir together the vinegar, Splenda, and the remaining 1 tablespoon curry powder. Pour the mixture over the pork. Cover the slow cooker, set it to low, and let it cook for 7 hours.

When the time's up, stir in the cauliflower. Re-cover the slow cooker and cook for 1 more hour, or until the cauliflower is tender.

YIELD: 6 servings, each with: 177 calories, 8 g fat, 17 g protein, 11 g carbohydrate, 3 g dietary fiber, 8 g usable carbs.

# Pork and "Apple" Stew

The apple flavor here comes from the apple cider vinegar. Our tester, Maria, cut her turnips into apple-slice shapes, and her family thought they were apples! They loved the whole thing.

2 pounds (1 kilogram) pork loin, cut into 1" cubes

2 medium turnips, cubed

2 medium carrots, cut 1/2" thick

1 medium onion, sliced

1/2 cup (60 grams) sliced celery

1 cup (235 milliliters) apple cider vinegar

3 tablespoons (4.5 grams) Splenda

1 cup (235 milliliters) chicken broth

1 teaspoon chicken bouillon concentrate

1 teaspoon caraway seeds

1/4 teaspoon pepper

Combine the pork, turnips, carrots, onion, and celery in your slow cooker.

In a bowl, stir together the vinegar, Splenda, broth, and bouillon. Pour the mixture over the pork and vegetables. Add the caraway seeds and pepper and stir everything. Cover the slow cooker, set it to low, and let it cook for 8 hours.

**YIELD:** 6 servings, each with: 226 calories, 6 g fat, 34 g protein, 10 g carbohydrate, 2 g dietary fiber, 8 g usable carbs.

# Easy Southwestern Pork Stew

Our tester gave this a 10—and so did her family!

1 medium onion, chopped

3 cloves garlic, crushed

2 pounds (1 kilogram) boneless pork loin, cut into 1" cubes

2 teaspoons ground cumin

1 tablespoon (4 grams) dried oregano

1/2 teaspoon salt

15 ounces (425 grams) canned black soybeans

14 1/2 ounces (411 grams) canned tomatoes with green chiles

1 cup (235 milliliters) chicken broth

1 teaspoon chicken bouillon concentrate

Put the onion and garlic in your slow cooker and place the pork on top.

In a bowl, stir together the cumin, oregano, salt, soybeans, tomatoes, broth, and bouillon. Pour the mixture over the pork and vegetables. Cover the slow cooker, set it to low, and let it cook for 8 to 9 hours.

**YIELD:** 6 servings, each with: 257 calories, 10 g fat, 34 g protein, 6 g carbohydrate, 1 g dietary fiber, 5 g usable carbs.

# Orange Pork Loin

Boneless pork loin frequently goes on sale. It's very lean, however, so it's often both bland and dry. Slow cooking takes care of that little problem! Sadly, fresh pumpkin is only available for a couple of months in the autumn, so that's when you'll need to make this dish. Buy a small pumpkin, or you'll have piles of it leftover.

1 pound (455 grams) pumpkin, peeled and cut into 1/2" cubes

1 pound (455 grams) rutabaga, cut into 1/2" cubes

2 tablespoons (28 milliliters) olive oil

2 pounds (1 kilogram) pork loin

2 tablespoons (40 grams) low-sugar marmalade or orange preserves

1/4 teaspoon orange extract

2 teaspoons Splenda

2 cloves garlic, crushed

1/2 teaspoon salt

1/2 cup (120 milliliters) chicken broth

Guar or xanthan

Put the pumpkin and rutabaga in the bottom of your slow cooker.

In a big, heavy skillet, heat the oil over medium-high heat and brown the pork all over. Put the pork in the slow cooker on top of the pumpkin and rutabaga.

In a bowl, stir together the marmalade, orange extract, Splenda, garlic, salt, and broth. Pour the mixture over the pork. Cover the slow cooker, set it to low, and let it cook for 8 hours.

When the time's up, carefully remove the pork to a platter and use a slotted spoon to pile the vegetables around it. Use guar or xanthan to thicken the liquid in the pot to the consistency of heavy cream. Serve the liquid with the pork and vegetables.

**YIELD:** 6 servings, each with: 281 calories, 10 g fat, 34 g protein, 13 g carbohydrate, 2 g dietary fiber, 11 g usable carbs.

# Pork Slow Cooker Chili

Try this when you want to have people over after the kids' soccer game!

1 tablespoon (14 milliliters) olive oil

2 1/2 pounds (1.25 kilograms) boneless pork loin, cut into 1" cubes

14 1/2 ounces (411 grams) canned tomatoes with green chiles

1/4 cup (25 grams) chopped onion

1/4 cup (30 grams) diced green bell pepper

1 clove garlic, crushed

1 tablespoon (7 grams) chili powder

In a big, heavy skillet, heat the oil and brown the pork all over. Transfer the pork to your slow cooker. Stir in the tomatoes, onion, pepper, garlic, and chili powder. Cover the slow cooker, set it to low, and let it cook for 6 to 8 hours.

Serve this with sour cream and shredded Monterey Jack cheese, if you like, but it's darned good as is.

**YIELD:** 8 servings, each with: 189 calories, 8 g fat, 25 g protein, 3 g carbohydrate, 1 g dietary fiber, 2 g usable carbs.

# Slow Cooker Mu Shu Pork

This isn't authentic, by any means, but it's very tasty. My husband, not a big Chinese food guy, really liked this.

2 plums, pitted and chopped

1 clove garlic, crushed

2 tablespoons (16 grams) grated ginger root

1/4 cup (60 milliliters) soy sauce

2 tablespoons (28 milliliters) dry sherry

2 teaspoons dark sesame oil

1/8 teaspoon five-spice powder

1 tablespoon (14 milliliters) rice vinegar

3 tablespoons (4.5 grams) Splenda

2 pounds (1 kilogram) boneless pork loin,
   cut into a few big chunks across the grain

Guar or xanthan

5 eggs, beaten

2 cups (100 grams) bean sprouts

2 cups (140 grams) shredded napa cabbage

16 6-inch low-carb tortillas

3/4 cup (75 grams) sliced scallions

Hoisin Sauce (optional, see recipe page 233)

Put the plums, garlic, ginger, soy sauce, sherry, sesame oil, five-spice powder, vinegar, and Splenda in a food processor with the S-blade in place and run until the plum is pureed.

Place the pork in your slow cooker. Pour the plum sauce over the pork. Cover the slow cooker, set it to low, and let it cook for 7 to 8 hours.

When the time's up, scoop out the pork with a slotted spoon and put it on a big plate. Use a couple of forks to tear the pork into little shreds. Thicken the sauce in the slow cooker to about ketchup consistency with guar or xanthan. Stir the shredded pork back into the slow cooker. Re-cover the slow cooker, set it to high, and let it cook for 30 minutes.

Meanwhile, spray a big, heavy skillet well with nonstick cooking spray. (A nonstick skillet is even better for this.) Put it over medium-high heat and let it get hot. Pour in enough of the eggs to form a thin layer on the bottom, and let it cook, not stirring, until it's a solid sheet. Lift the eggs out and set them on a plate. Cook the rest of the eggs into a thin sheet, as well. Use a sharp knife to cut these sheets of cooked egg into strips about 1/4" (5 millimeters) wide. Reserve.

When the 30 minutes are up, stir the bean sprouts, cabbage, and shredded eggs into the pork mixture. Re-cover the slow cooker and let it cook for just another 10 to 15 minutes. (You want the bean sprouts to be hot through, but still have some crispness.) While that's happening, slice your scallions. (If you're not going to be eating all of this right away, only slice enough scallions for immediate use.)

To serve, spread 1/3 cup of the pork-and-egg-and-vegetable mixture on a tortilla, sprinkle with sliced scallions, wrap, and eat! If you want to be more authentic, you could spread a little Hoisin Sauce on each tortilla before filling, but it's hardly essential.

**YIELD:** 16 servings, each with: 175 calories, 8 g fat, 19 g protein, 14 g carbohydrate, 9 g dietary fiber, 5 g usable carbs.

# Hot Asian Ribs

This is full-bodied Chinese flavor. If your family loves Chinese spareribs, you have to make this!

3 1/2 pounds (1.75 kilograms) country-style pork ribs

4 scallions, sliced

1/4 cup (60 milliliters) soy sauce

1/3 cup (8 grams) Splenda

1 teaspoon blackstrap molasses

2 tablespoons (28 milliliters) white wine vinegar

2 teaspoons toasted sesame oil

2 teaspoons lemon juice

1/2 teaspoon hot sauce

1 clove garlic

1/2 teaspoon ground ginger

1/2 teaspoon chili powder

1/4 teaspoon red pepper flakes

6 teaspoons Hoisin Sauce (see recipe page 233)

Put the ribs in your slow cooker.

In a bowl, mix together the scallions, soy sauce, Splenda, molasses, vinegar, sesame oil, lemon juice, hot sauce, garlic, ginger, chili powder, red pepper flakes, and Hoisin Sauce. Pour the sauce over the ribs. Cover the slow cooker, set it to low, and let it cook for 8 to 9 hours.

**YIELD:** 6 servings, each with: 469 calories, 35 g fat, 32 g protein, 4 g carbohydrate, 1 g dietary fiber, 3 g usable carbs.

# ⊡ Key West Ribs

Citrusy barbecue sauce gives this a Florida kind of taste!

3 pounds (1.5 kilograms) country-style pork ribs

1/4 cup (30 grams) finely chopped onion

1/4 cup (60 milliliters) low-carb barbecue sauce
(recipe from page 231 or purchased)

1 teaspoon grated orange peel

1 teaspoon grated lemon rind

1/2 teaspoon salt

2 tablespoons (28 milliliters) white wine vinegar

2 tablespoons (28 milliliters) lemon juice

2 tablespoons (28 milliliters) lime juice

1 1/2 tablespoons (2 grams) Splenda

1/8 teaspoon orange extract

2 tablespoons (28 milliliters) olive oil

In a big, heavy skillet, brown the ribs over medium-high heat. Transfer them to your slow cooker.

In a bowl, mix together the onion, barbecue sauce, orange peel, lemon rind, salt, vinegar, lemon juice, lime juice, Splenda, orange extract, and oil. Pour the mixture over the ribs. Cover the slow cooker, set it to low, and let it cook for 7 to 9 hours.

Serve the ribs together with the sauce.

YIELD: 6 servings, each with: 421 calories, 33 g fat, 26 g protein, 3 g carbohydrate, trace dietary fiber, 3 g usable carbs.

# Maple-Spice Country-Style Ribs

My pal Ray Stevens, who has tested many recipes for me, raves about this. It's shaping up to be the recipe by which all other recipes are judged!

3 pounds (1.5 kilograms) country-style pork ribs

1/2 cup (120 milliliters) sugar-free pancake syrup

3 tablespoons (4.5 grams) Splenda

2 tablespoons (28 milliliters) soy sauce

1/4 cup (25 grams) chopped onion

1/2 teaspoon ground cinnamon

1/2 teaspoon ground ginger

1/2 teaspoon ground allspice

3 cloves garlic, crushed

1/4 teaspoon pepper

1/8 teaspoon cayenne

Put the ribs in your slow cooker.

In a bowl, mix together the syrup, Splenda, soy sauce, onion, cinnamon, ginger, allspice, garlic, pepper, and cayenne. Pour the mixture over the ribs. Cover the slow cooker, set it to low, and let it cook for 9 hours.

**YIELD:** 6 servings, each with: 382 calories, 29 g fat, 27 g protein, 2 g carbohydrate, trace dietary fiber, 2 g usable carbs.

# Orange-Glazed Country Ribs

Fruit flavors of all kinds bring out the best in pork.

2 pounds (1 kilograms) boneless pork country-style ribs

1/2 small onion, sliced

1 clove garlic, crushed

1/2 tablespoon (7 grams) butter

1/2 cup (60 grams) finely chopped green bell pepper

1/2 clove garlic, crushed

3 tablespoons (60 grams) low-sugar orange marmalade

1/4 cup (60 milliliters) lemon juice

1 tablespoon (1.5 grams) Splenda

1/4 teaspoon orange extract

1 tablespoon (8 grams) grated ginger root

Guar or xanthan

Spray your slow cooker with nonstick cooking spray. Add the ribs, onion, and garlic. Cover the slow cooker, set it to low, and let it cook for 7 to 8 hours.

When the time's up, melt the butter in a medium-size nonreactive saucepan. Add the pepper and garlic and sauté until it's just soft. Add the marmalade, lemon juice, Splenda, orange extract, and ginger, bring to a simmer, and let it cook for 5 minutes. Thicken the sauce a little with guar or xanthan.

Remove the ribs from the slow cooker and put them on a broiler rack. Brush them with the sauce and run them under the broiler, set on high, for 5 minutes to glaze. Serve with the rest of the sauce.

**YIELD:** 6 servings, each with: 304 calories, 20 g fat, 27 g protein, 3 g carbohydrate, trace dietary fiber, 3 g usable carbs.

# Ribs 'n' Kraut

If you like, you can make this with smoked sausage instead of the country-style ribs. If you do, read the labels to find the lowest carb smoked sausage.

2 pounds (1 kilogram) country-style pork ribs

1 medium Granny Smith apple, diced

1/2 medium onion, sliced

16 ounces (455 grams) sauerkraut, rinsed and drained

3 tablespoons (4.5 grams) Splenda

1/2 teaspoon blackstrap molasses

1 teaspoon caraway seeds

1/4 cup (60 milliliters) dry white wine

Put the ribs, apple, and onion in your slow cooker. Cover with the sauerkraut.

In a bowl, stir together the Splenda, molasses, caraway seeds, and wine. Pour the mixture over the sauerkraut and ribs. Cover the slow cooker, set it to low, and let it cook for 8 hours.

**YIELD:** 6 servings, each with: 286 calories, 19 g fat, 18 g protein, 7 g carbohydrate, 3 g dietary fiber, 4 g usable carbs.

# Ribs with Apple Kraut

Even folks who aren't wild about sauerkraut may like this. With the apple and the other vegetables, there's a lot more than just sauerkraut going on here.

3 1/2 pounds (1.75 kilograms) country-style pork ribs

2 tablespoons (28 milliliters) oil

3/4 cup (110 grams) diced cauliflower

3/4 cup (110 grams) diced turnip

1 Granny Smith apple, cored and thinly sliced

2 carrots, sliced

1 medium onion, sliced

1 pound (455 grams) sauerkraut, rinsed and drained

1/2 cup (120 milliliters) apple cider vinegar

3 tablespoons (4.5 grams) Splenda

2 teaspoons caraway seeds

1/8 teaspoon ground cloves

Guar or xanthan

In a big, heavy skillet, brown the ribs in the oil over medium-high heat.

Put the cauliflower, turnip, apple, carrots, and onion in your slow cooker. Put the ribs and sauerkraut on top.

In a bowl, mix together the vinegar, Splenda, caraway seeds, and cloves. Pour the mixture over the ribs and sauerkraut. Cover the slow cooker, set it to low, and let it cook for 8 to 9 hours.

When the time's up, remove the ribs to a platter with tongs and scoop out the vegetables with a slotted spoon. Thicken the pot liquid with guar or xanthan, add salt and pepper to taste, and serve the sauce with the ribs and vegetables.

**YIELD:** 6 servings, each with: 529 calories, 39 g fat, 32 g protein, 13 g carbohydrate, 4 g dietary fiber, 9 g usable carbs.

# ▢ Slow Cooker Barbecue

This is simple, simple, simple.

> 2 tablespoons (12 grams) Classic Rub (see recipe page 234)
>> or prepared spice rub
>
> 2 1/2 pounds (1.25 kilograms) pork spareribs, cut into 2 or 3 pieces
>> to fit into your slow cooker
>
> 1/3 cup (75 milliliters) Dana's "Kansas City" Barbecue Sauce
>> (see recipe page 231) or purchased low-carb barbecue sauce

Sprinkle 1 tablespoon of rub over each side of the ribs. Put the ribs on a broiler rack and broil them on high, about 6" (15 centimeters) from the heat, for about 5 to 7 minutes per side, or until well browned. Transfer the ribs to your slow cooker.

Pour the barbecue sauce evenly over the ribs and use a spoon to spread it, so the "up" side of the ribs is coated. Cover the slow cooker, set it to low, and let it cook for 6 hours.

**YIELD:** 3 servings, each with: 688 calories, 56 g fat, 40 g protein, 4 g carbohydrate, trace dietary fiber, 4 g usable carbs.

# Polynesian Pork Ribs

It's a luau in your slow cooker!

2 pounds (1 kilogram) country-style pork ribs

1 clove garlic, crushed

1/2 medium onion, sliced

1/4 cup (50 grams) canned crushed pineapple in juice

1/2 cup (120 grams) Dana's No-Sugar Ketchup (see recipe page 228)
   or purchased low-carb ketchup

1 tablespoon (1.5 grams) Splenda

1/2 teaspoon blackstrap molasses

1 tablespoon (14 milliliters) soy sauce

1 teaspoon grated ginger root

1/2 teaspoon dark sesame oil

1 tablespoon (14 milliliters) cider vinegar

Put the ribs in your slow cooker, along with the garlic and onion.

In a bowl, stir together the pineapple and 1/4 cup of the ketchup. Pour the mixture over the ribs. Cover the slow cooker, set it to low, and let it cook for 8 to 10 hours.

When the time's up, pull the ribs out of the slow cooker, put them on a broiler rack, and stash them somewhere warm.

Ladle the cooking liquid into a saucepan. Stir in the remaining 1/4 cup ketchup, the Splenda, molasses, soy sauce, ginger, sesame oil, and vinegar, bring to a simmer, and let cook until you have a passably thick sauce.

Spoon the sauce over the ribs and run them under the broiler for 5 minutes or so, just to glaze them a bit.

YIELD: 6 servings, each with: 288 calories, 20 g fat, 19 g protein, 9 g carbohydrate, 1 g dietary fiber, 8 g usable carbs.

# Soy and Sesame Ribs

Here's another Asian take on ribs. The toasted sesame seed topping really sets this recipe apart.

3 pounds (1.5 kilograms) pork spareribs

1/3 cup (8 grams) Splenda

1/4 cup (60 grams) Dana's No-Sugar Ketchup (see recipe page 228)

    or prepared low-carb ketchup

1 tablespoon (20 grams) sugar-free imitation honey

1 tablespoon (28 milliliters) cider vinegar

1 clove garlic, crushed

1/2 teaspoon ground ginger

1/2 teaspoon red pepper flakes

1/2 teaspoon dark sesame oil

1 tablespoon (8 grams) sesame seeds

4 scallions, thinly sliced

Cut the ribs into portions if needed to fit them in your slow cooker. Broil the ribs about 6" (16 centimeters) from high heat until browned, about 10 minutes per side. Transfer them to your slow cooker.

In a bowl, mix together the Splenda, ketchup, honey, vinegar, garlic, ginger, red pepper, and sesame oil. Pour the mixture over the ribs, turning to coat if needed. Cover the slow cooker, set it to low, and let it cook for 5 to 6 hours.

Toast the sesame seeds by stirring them in a dry skillet over medium-high heat until they start to make popping sounds and jump around a bit. Serve the ribs with sesame seeds and scallions scattered over them.

**YIELD:** 4 servings, each with: 646 calories, 52 g fat, 37 g protein, 7 g carbohydrate, 1 g dietary fiber, 6 g usable carbs. (Counts do not include the polyols in the imitation honey.)

# Teriyaki-Tangerine Ribs

This is an easy twist on plain old teriyaki.

  4 pounds (2 kilograms) country-style pork ribs
  Teriyaki Sauce (see recipe page 233)
  Florida Sunshine Tangerine Barbecue Sauce (see recipe page 230)

Put the ribs in your slow cooker.

In a bowl, mix together the Teriyaki Sauce and the Florida Sunshine Tangerine Barbecue Sauce. Pour the mixture over the ribs. Cover the slow cooker, set it to low, and let it cook for 7 to 8 hours.

When the time's up, remove the ribs. Transfer the sauce to a nonreactive saucepan and put it over high heat. Boil it hard until it thickens up a bit and serve the sauce over the ribs.

**YIELD:** 8 servings, each with: 415 calories, 29 g fat, 28 g protein, 8 g carbohydrate, 1 g dietary fiber, 7 g usable carbs.

# Slow Cooker Pulled Pork

Pulled pork is a Carolina tradition, and it usually involves many, many hours of long, slow smoking. This is not authentic, but it is tasty, and thanks to liquid smoke flavoring, it has an appealingly smoky flavor. This recipe requires a meat injector, a big, scary-looking syringe that looks like your doctor got way out of hand. You can buy inexpensive ones at housewares stores.

1/3 cup (75 milliliters) liquid smoke flavoring

3 pounds (1.5 kilograms) pork shoulder

Sauces, such as Eastern Carolina Vinegar Sauce (see recipe page 232),
   Dana's "Kansas City" Barbecue Sauce (see recipe page 231),
   and Piedmont Mustard Sauce (see recipe page 232)

Slurp up a syringe-full of the liquid smoke flavoring and inject it into a dozen sites all over the pork shoulder. Season the pork with salt and pepper. Place the pork in your slow cooker and pour another tablespoon or two of liquid smoke over it. Cover the slow cooker, set it to low, and let it cook for 8 hours.

When the time's up, remove the pork from the slow cooker and pull out the bone, which will be very easy to do at this point. Discard the bone, along with any surface fat. Use two forks to pull the meat into shreds. Toss it with one of the sauces.

You can serve Pulled Pork in one of a few ways: You can wrap it in low-carb tortillas, serve it on low-carb buns, or, my favorite, serve it on a bed of coleslaw.

**YIELD:** 6 servings, each with: 405 calories, 31 g fat, 29 g protein, trace carbohydrate, trace dietary fiber, 0 g usable carbs.

# Slow Cooker Teriyaki Ribs

This dish is sweet, spicy, and tangy, and falling-off-the-bone tender

> 6 pounds (3 kilograms) pork spareribs, cut into 3 or 4 pieces so they fit in the
> slow cooker
> 3/4 cup (180 grams) Dana's No-Sugar Ketchup (see recipe page 228)
> or purchased low-carb ketchup
> 1 batch Teriyaki Sauce (see recipe page 233)
> 1/4 cup (6 grams) Splenda
> 1/4 teaspoon blackstrap molasses
> 1 teaspoon minced garlic or 2 cloves garlic, crushed
> Guar or xanthan

Place the ribs in your slow cooker.

In a bowl, mix the ketchup, Teriyaki Sauce, Splenda, molasses, and garlic together.
Pour the mixture over the ribs. Cover the slow cooker, set it to low, and let it cook for
10 hours.

When the time's up, use tongs to pull out the now unbelievably tender and flavorful
ribs. Ladle out as much of the pot liquid as you think you'll use and thicken it using
guar or xanthan. Serve the sauce over the ribs.

**YIELD:** 8 servings, each with: 650 calories, 50 g fat, 38 g protein, 9 g carbohydrate,
1 g dietary fiber (depending on how much of the liquid you eat), about 8 g usable carbs.

# Fruity, Spicy Ribs

This recipe is a little hot, a little sweet, a little Southwestern, and a little Asian—but all tasty.

6 pounds (3 kilograms) pork spareribs, cut in pieces so they fit in your slow cooker

6 tablespoons (120 grams) low-sugar apricot preserves

1/3 cup (75 milliliters) lemon juice

2 tablespoons (3 grams) Splenda

2 tablespoons (15 grams) chili powder

2 teaspoons five-spice powder

1/4 cup (60 milliliters) soy sauce

1/2 cup (120 milliliters) chicken broth

Put the ribs on a broiler rack and broil them about 6" (15 centimeters) from high heat for about 7 to 8 minutes per side, or until browned. Transfer the ribs to your slow cooker.

In a bowl, mix together the preserves, lemon juice, Splenda, chili powder, five-spice powder, soy sauce, and broth. Pour the mixture over the ribs. Cover the slow cooker, set it to low, and let it cook for 6 to 7 hours.

When the time's up, remove the ribs to a platter. Pour off the liquid in the pot into a deep, clear container, and let the fat rise to the top. Skim off the fat. Now pour the liquid into a saucepan. Boil it hard until it's reduced by at least half and starting to thicken. Serve the sauce with the ribs.

YIELD: 8 servings, each with: 636 calories, 50 g fat, 37 g protein, 7 g carbohydrate, 1 g dietary fiber, 6 g usable carbs.

# Rosemary-Ginger Ribs with Apricot Glaze

This recipe originally appeared in *15-Minute Low-Carb Recipes*. Feel free to use a full-size slab of ribs—about 6 pounds (3 kilograms) worth—and double the seasonings if you're feeding a family.

1 slab baby back ribs, about 2 1/2 pounds (about 1 kilogram)

Rosemary-ginger rub (I use a brand called Stubb's.)

2 tablespoons (40 grams) low-sugar apricot preserves

1 1/2 teaspoons spicy brown mustard

1 teaspoon Splenda

1 1/2 teaspoons soy sauce

Sprinkle both sides of the ribs generously with the rosemary-ginger rub. Curl the slab of ribs around and fit it down into your slow cooker. Cover the slow cooker, set it to low, and let it cook for 9 to 10 hours. (No, I didn't forget anything. You don't put any liquid in the slow cooker. Don't sweat it.)

When the time's up, mix together the preserves, mustard, Splenda, and soy sauce. Carefully remove the ribs from the slow cooker. (They may fall apart on you a bit because they'll be so tender.) Arrange the ribs meaty-side-up on a broiler rack. Spread the apricot glaze evenly over the ribs and run them under a broiler set on high, 3 to 4 inches (7 to 10 centimeters) from the heat, for 7 to 8 minutes.

**YIELD:** 3 servings, each with: 689 calories, 56 g fat, 40 g protein, 4 g carbohydrate, trace dietary fiber, 4 g usable carbs.

# Slow Cooker "Barbecued" Ribs

Okay, it's not really barbecue because it's not done over a fire. But this recipe tastes great and lets you dig into your ribs within minutes of walking in the door.

> 2 1/2 pounds (about 1 kilogram) pork spare ribs
> 2 tablespons (15 grams) Classic Rub (see recipe page 234) or purchased dry rub
> 1/3 cup (150 milliliters) Dana's "Kansas City" Barbecue Sauce (see recipe page 231) or purchased low-carb barbecue sauce

Sprinkle the slab of ribs liberally on both sides with the dry rub, coil the ribs up, and slide them into your slow cooker. Cover the slow cooker, set it to low, and let it cook for 9 to 10 hours.

When the time's up, pull the ribs out of the slow cooker. (Do this carefully because they'll be falling-apart tender.) Lay the ribs on a broiler rack, meaty-side-up, and spread the barbecue sauce over them. Broil 3 to 4 inches (7 to 10 centimeters) from the broiler set on high for 7 to 8 minutes.

**NOTE:** If you'd like to give these a smoked flavor, you can buy liquid smoke flavoring at your grocery store. Simply brush the ribs with the liquid smoke before you sprinkle on the dry rub.

**YIELD:** 3 servings, each with: 688 calories, 56 g fat, 40 g protein, 4 g carbohydrate, 1 g dietary fiber, 3 g usable carbs. (Your carb count will be a bit different depending on whether you use homemade sugar-free barbecue sauce or commercial low-carb sauce.)

# About Pork Neckbones

Unless you grew up on soul food, you may never have tried pork neckbones. They're another one of those cuts that are perfect for the slow cooker. They're bony and tough, and cheap. My grocery store has them for 59 cents a pound week in and week out. Yet cooked with slow moist heat, they're incredibly flavorful, and because the meat falls right off the bone, who cares that they're bony?

I did have one teeny problem with pork neckbones: I simply could not find any nutritional statistics for them, and I even wrote to a big pork producer! However, you can count on them being carb-free, so these carb counts are accurate. It's the protein and calorie counts that I couldn't get, so that's why they're missing in these neckbone recipes.

## Stewed Pork Neckbones with Turnips and Cabbage

This one-pot meal is not a beautiful dish to look at, but boy, does it taste good! Plenty of Tabasco is essential.

3 turnips, diced
3 pounds (1.5 kilograms) meaty pork neckbones
1 teaspoon red pepper flakes
1 1/2 teaspoons salt or Vege-Sal
3 cups (705 milliliters) water
1/2 head cabbage, cut in wedges
Tabasco sauce

Put the turnips in the bottom of your slow cooker. Put the neckbones on top of them. Sprinkle the red pepper and salt or Vege-Sal over it, then pour the water over that. Now arrange the cabbage wedges on top of that. Cover the slow cooker, set it to low, and let it cook for 7 to 8 hours.

Scoop everything out onto a platter together with a slotted spoon and dose it well with Tabasco sauce before serving.

**YIELD:** 4 servings, each with: 6 g carbohydrate, 2 g dietary fiber, 4 g usable carbs.

# Neckbones and "Rice"

I adapted this recipe from one on a soul food Web site. I have no experience with genuine soul food, so I can't tell you how close this comes, but it's great in its own right.

2 1/2 pounds (1.25 kilograms) meaty pork neckbones

1/2 cup (120 milliliters) oil

1 medium onion, sliced

1 tablespoon (9 grams) garlic powder

1 teaspoon salt or Vege-Sal

1 teaspoon pepper

2 cups (475 milliliters) chicken broth

1/2 head cauliflower

Guar or xanthan

In a big, heavy skillet, brown the pork neckbones in the oil over medium-high heat, in batches. Transfer the neckbones to your slow cooker.

Add the onion and sprinkle the garlic powder, salt or Vege-Sal, and pepper over the whole thing. Pour in the broth and give the whole thing a stir. Cover the slow cooker, set it to low, and let it cook for 6 to 7 hours.

When the time's up, run the cauliflower through the shredding blade of a food processor. Put the resulting Cauli-Rice in a microwaveable casserole dish with a lid. Add a couple of tablespoons of water, cover, and microwave on high for 7 minutes.

Meanwhile, remove the neckbones to a platter. Thicken the liquid a little with guar or xanthan. Serve the neckbones, onions, and gravy over the Cauli-Rice.

**YIELD:** 3 servings, each with: 7 g carbohydrate, 1 g dietary fiber, 6 g usable carbs.

# Cocido de Puerco

This pork stew appeared in *500 Low-Carb Recipes*, but I hadn't thought of slow cooking it yet. It worked out great!

- 3 pounds (1.5 kilograms) pork neckbones
- 2 tablespoons (28 milliliters) olive oil
- 1 small onion, chopped
- 1 clove garlic, crushed
- 1 green bell pepper, diced
- 2 medium zucchini, chunked
- 14 1/2 ounces (411 grams) canned diced tomatoes
- 2 teaspoons cumin
- 2 teaspoons dried oregano
- 1/2 teaspoon red pepper flakes
- 1 large onion, sliced

In a big, heavy skillet, brown the pork neckbones in the oil.

While that's happening, put the onion and garlic in the bottom of your slow cooker. When the neckbones are browned, put them in the slow cooker on top of the onions. Put the pepper and zucchini on top.

In a bowl, stir together the tomatoes, cumin, oregano, and red pepper. Pour the mixture into the slow cooker. Cover the slow cooker, set it to low, and let it cook for 6 to 7 hours.

**YIELD:** 5 servings, each with: 12 g carbohydrate, 2 g dietary fiber, 10 g usable carbs.

# Stuffed Peppers

6 large green peppers

1 1/2 pounds (700 grams) bulk Italian sausage

1/2 head cauliflower

2 cups (500 grams) no-sugar-added spaghetti sauce

2/3 cup (110 grams) crumbled feta cheese

1/2 cup (50 grams) chopped onion

1/4 cup (40 grams) chopped tomato

1/4 cup (16 grams) chopped fresh parsley

2 tablespoons (12 grams) chopped black olives

1 clove garlic, crushed

1/2 teaspoon salt or Vege-Sal

1 teaspoon Italian seasoning

1/2 teaspoon red pepper flakes

Cut the tops off the peppers. Remove the usable pepper wall from the stems and chop it, discarding the stems and seeds. Reserve the pepper shells.

In a big, heavy skillet, brown and crumble the sausage till done. Drain the fat.

Run the cauliflower through the shredding blade of a food processor. Place the resulting Cauli-Rice in a big mixing bowl.

Put 1 cup of the spaghetti sauce in the slow cooker. Add the rest to the Cauli-Rice. Add the cheese, onion, tomato, parsley, olives, garlic, salt or Vege-Sal, Italian seasoning, red pepper, cooked sausage, and the chopped bit of green pepper to the Cauli-Rice. Combine well. Divide the mixture between the pepper shells.

Put the stuffed peppers in the slow cooker. Cover the slow cooker, set it to low, and let it cook for 4 to 5 hours, or until the peppers are tender.

YIELD: 6 servings, each with: 592 calories, 51 g fat, 18 g protein, 18 g carbohydrate, 5 g dietary fiber, 13 g usable carbs.

# Tangy Pork Chops

4 pounds (2 kilograms) pork chops, 1/2" thick

1/2 teaspoon salt or Vege-Sal

1/4 teaspoon pepper

1/2 cup (50 grams) chopped onion

2 stalks celery, diced

1 green bell pepper, diced

14 1/2 ounces (411 grams) canned diced tomatoes

1/2 cup (120 grams) Dana's No-Sugar Ketchup (see recipe page 228)
    or purchased low-carb ketchup

2 tablespoons (28 milliliters) cider vinegar

2 tablespoons (30 grams) Worcestershire sauce

2 tablespoons (3 grams) Splenda

1/4 teaspoon blackstrap molasses

1 tablespoon (14 milliliters) lemon juice

1 teaspoon beef bouillon concentrate

Guar or xanthan

Place the pork in the bottom of your slow cooker. Sprinkle the pork with the salt and pepper. Now add the onion, celery, green pepper, and tomatoes.

In a bowl, stir together the ketchup, vinegar, Worcestershire sauce, Splenda, molasses, lemon juice, and bouillon. Stir until the bouillon dissolves. Pour the mixture into the slow cooker. Cover the slow cooker, set it to low, and let it cook for 5 to 6 hours.

When the time's up, remove the pork and place it on a platter. Use a slotted spoon to pile the vegetables around the pork. Thicken the liquid left in the slow cooker with guar or xanthan and serve the sauce with the pork and vegetables.

**YIELD:** 8 servings, each with: 396 calories, 23 g fat, 36 g protein, 11 g carbohydrate, 1 g dietary fiber, 10 g usable carbs.

# Onion-Mustard Pork Chops

2 pounds (1 kilogram) pork chops

1 tablespoon (14 milliliters) olive oil

1 medium onion, thinly sliced

4 cloves garlic, crushed

1 teaspoon dry mustard

1/2 teaspoon salt or Vege-Sal

1 teaspoon pepper

1 dash hot sauce

1 tablespoon (14 milliliters) cider vinegar

1/2 cup (120 milliliters) dry white wine

2 tablespoons (30 grams) brown mustard

1/2 cup (120 milliliters) heavy cream

Guar or xanthan

In a big, heavy skillet, brown the pork on both sides in the oil over medium-high heat. Transfer the pork to your slow cooker.

Turn the heat down to medium-low and add the onion to the skillet. Sauté it until it's translucent. Then stir in the garlic, dry mustard, salt or Vege-Sal, pepper, and hot sauce and let the whole thing sauté for another minute or so. Transfer the mixture to the slow cooker on top of the pork.

In a bowl, stir together the vinegar and wine. Pour the mixture into the slow cooker. Cover the slow cooker, set it to low, and let it cook for 6 hours.

When the time's up, remove the pork to a platter. Stir the mustard and cream into the juice in the pot. Thicken the juice a tad with guar or xanthan and serve the sauce over the pork.

**YIELD:** 6 servings, each with: 352 calories, 25 g fat, 25 g protein, 4 g carbohydrate, 1 g dietary fiber, 3 g usable carbs.

# Choucroute Garni

This is a streamlined version of a traditional dish from the Alsace region of France. The name means Garnished Sauerkraut. It's so simple and so good, especially on a cold night.

    14 ounces (400 grams) canned sauerkraut, rinsed and drained

    1 tablespoon (14 milliliters) bacon grease

    1/4 cup (60 milliliters) apple cider vinegar

    1 tablespoon (1.5 grams) Splenda

    1/2 medium onion, thinly sliced

    2 tablespoons (28 milliliters) gin

    1/4 cup (60 milliliters) dry white wine

    1 pound (455 grams) meat (Choose any combination of kielbasa, smoked
        sausage, frankfurters, link sausages, 1/4-inch-thick (5 millimeter)
        ham slices, or smoked pork chops.*)

Place the sauerkraut in your slow cooker. Add the bacon grease, vinegar, Splenda, onion, gin, and wine and give it a quick stir. Place the meat on top. Cover the slow cooker, set it to low, and let it cook for 5 to 6 hours.

*I use 1/2 pound (225 g) each of the lowest carbohydrate kielbasa and smoked sausage I can find.

NOTE: This doesn't even start to fill my slow cooker, so feel free to double or even triple this recipe. If you increase it, I suggest arranging it with a layer of kraut, a layer of meat, a layer of kraut, and so on. And, of course, you'll have to increase the cooking time by an hour, maybe two, depending on how many extra layers you use.

YIELD: 3 servings, each with: 112 calories, 5 g fat, 1 g protein, 9 g carbohydrate, 4 g dietary fiber, 5 g usable carbs. (This will depend on which meats you use.)

# CHAPTER SIX

# Slow Cooker Lamb

You'll notice a certain reliance on lamb shanks here. Lamb shanks are the bottom-most part of a leg of lamb, and they're ideal for slow cooking for a couple reasons. They fit neatly in the pot, and they're the sort of tough, flavorful meat that really shines with slow, moist cooking.

If you're having trouble finding lamb shanks at your grocery store, ask the nice meat guys. Or you could make any of the shank recipes with a chunk of lamb leg or shoulder of the right weight. Have the meat guys cut it into a few pieces, though, so it'll fit in your pot and won't take far more cooking time than the recipe specifies. Most grocery stores will cut up a roast for you for no added charge.

# Lamb Shanks in Red Wine

This is a hearty one-pot meal.

5 pounds (2.5 kilograms) lamb shank (4 shanks)
1/4 cup (60 milliliters) olive oil
2 stalks celery, sliced 1/2" thick
2 carrots, sliced 1/2" thick
8 cloves garlic, crushed
1/2 onion, chunked
8 ounces (225 grams) sliced mushrooms
1 cup (235 milliliters) chicken broth
1 cup (235 milliliters) dry red wine
1 teaspoon beef bouillon concentrate
2 teaspoons pepper
1/2 teaspoon ground rosemary
2 bay leaves
Guar or xanthan

In a big, heavy skillet, sear the lamb all over in the oil.

Place the celery, carrots, garlic, onion, and mushrooms in your slow cooker.

When the lamb is browned all over, transfer it to the slow cooker, on top of the veggies.

In a bowl, stir together the broth, wine, bouillon, pepper, and rosemary. Pour the mixture over the lamb. Add the bay leaves. (Make sure they land in the liquid!) Cover the slow cooker, turn it to low, and let it cook for 6 hours.

When the time's up, remove the lamb to serving plates. Using guar or xanthan, thicken the liquid in the slow cooker to the consistency of heavy cream. Ladle the sauce and vegetables over the lamb.

**YIELD:** 6 servings, each with: 757 calories, 50 g fat, 59 g protein, 8 g carbohydrate, 2 g dietary fiber, 6 g usable carbs.

# Lemon Lamb Shanks

Lemon brings out the best in lamb!

4 pounds (2 kilograms) lamb shank

2 tablespoons (28 milliliters) olive oil

1 teaspoon lemon pepper

1/2 teaspoon dry mustard

1/2 cup (120 milliliters) chicken broth

1 teaspoon beef bouillon concentrate

1/2 teaspoon grated lemon peel

2 tablespoons (28 milliliters) lemon juice

1 teaspoon dried rosemary

2 cloves garlic, crushed

Guar or xanthan

Sear the lamb all over in the oil. Place the lamb in your slow cooker.

In a bowl, mix together the lemon pepper and dry mustard. Sprinkle the mixture evenly over the lamb.

In the same bowl, mix together the broth, bouillon, lemon peel, lemon juice, rosemary, and garlic. Pour the mixture over the lamb. Cover the slow cooker, set it to low, and let it cook for 8 hours.

When the time's up, remove the lamb and thicken up the liquid in the slow cooker a bit with guar or xanthan.

Serve this dish with a salad with plenty of cucumbers and tomatoes!

**YIELD:** 6 servings, each with: 535 calories, 37 g fat, 46 g protein, 1 g carbohydrate, trace dietary fiber, 1 g usable carbs.

# Kashmiri Lamb Shanks

This was originally a recipe for a skillet curry of lamb, but it works wonderfully in the slow cooker. If you like Indian food, you have to try this. And if you've never eaten Indian food, you need to start!

2 1/2 pounds (1.25 kilograms) lamb shank

2 tablespoons (28 milliliters) olive oil

1 cup (235 milliliters) chicken broth

1/2 teaspoon beef bouillon concentrate

1 teaspoon Garam Masala (see recipe page 236) or purchased garam masala

2 teaspoons ground coriander

1 tablespoon (8 grams) grated ginger root

1/4 teaspoon cayenne

Guar or xanthan

In a big, heavy skillet, sear the lamb all over in the oil over medium-high heat. Transfer the lamb to your slow cooker.

In a bowl, mix together the broth, bouillon, garam masala, coriander, ginger, and cayenne. Pour the mixture over the lamb. Cover the slow cooker, set it to low, and let it cook for 8 hours.

Remove the lamb to a platter, thicken the sauce a bit with guar or xanthan, and serve the sauce over the lamb.

YIELD: 4 servings, each with: 530 calories, 38 g fat, 44 g protein, 1 g carbohydrate, trace dietary fiber, 1 g usable carbs.

# Seriously Simple Lamb Shanks

Simple is good!

> 3 pounds (1.5 kilograms) lamb shank
>
> 2 tablespoons (28 milliliters) olive oil
>
> 1 cup (235 milliliters) chicken broth
>
> 1 teaspoon beef bouillon concentrate
>
> 2 teaspoons paprika
>
> 5 cloves garlic, crushed
>
> Guar or xanthan

Season the lamb all over with salt and pepper. In a big, heavy skillet, over medium-high heat, sear the lamb in the oil until it's brown all over. Transfer the lamb to your slow cooker.

In a bowl, mix together the broth and bouillon. Pour the mixture over the lamb. Sprinkle the paprika and garlic over the lamb. Cover the slow cooker, set it to low, and let it cook for 6 to 7 hours.

Remove the lamb with tongs and put it on a serving plate. Pour the liquid in the slow cooker into a 2-cup glass measuring cup and let the fat rise to the top. Skim the fat off and discard, and then thicken up the remaining liquid using guar or xanthan. Serve the sauce with the shanks.

Either Cauli-Rice (see recipe page 239) or Fauxtatoes (see recipe page 239) would be nice with this, but it's fine with just a simple salad or vegetable side.

**YIELD:** 4 servings, each with: 627 calories, 44 g fat, 52 g protein, 2 g carbohydrate, trace dietary fiber, 2 g usable carbs.

# Lamb Stew Provençal

I turned this recipe over to my sister to test. She's mad for French food, especially from Provence. She gave this the thumbs-up.

3 pounds (1.5 kilograms) lamb stew meat—shoulder is good, cubed. (Have the meat guys cut it off the bone.)

3 tablespoons (45 milliliters) olive oil

1 whole fennel bulb, sliced lengthwise

1 medium onion, sliced lengthwise

4 cloves garlic, crushed

1 bay leaf

1 teaspoon dried rosemary, whole needles

15 ounces (425 grams) canned black soybeans, drained

1 cup (235 milliliters) beef broth

1 teaspoon chicken bouillon concentrate

1/2 teaspoon dried basil

1/2 teaspoon dried marjoram

1/2 teaspoon dried savory

1/2 teaspoon dried thyme

Guar or xanthan

Season the lamb with salt and pepper. In a big, heavy skillet, heat the oil and brown the lamb on all sides over medium-high heat.

Place the fennel, onion, and garlic in the bottom of your slow cooker. Add the bay leaf and rosemary. Dump the soybeans on top of that. When the lamb is browned, put it on top of the vegetables.

In a bowl, stir together the broth, bouillon, basil, marjoram, savory, and thyme. Pour the mixture over the lamb. Cover the slow cooker, set it to low, and let it cook for 8 to 9 hours.

When it's done, thicken the liquid to the texture of heavy cream with guar or xanthan.

**YIELD:** 8 servings, each with: 348 calories, 17 g fat, 41 g protein, 8 g carbohydrate, 4 g dietary fiber, 4 g usable carbs.

# Caribbean Slow Cooker Lamb

Lamb and goat are very popular in the Caribbean, and this is my slow cooker interpretation of a Caribbean lamb dish. Look for tamarind concentrate in a grocery store with a good international section. I found it in a medium-size town in southern Indiana, so you may well find it near you! If you can't find it, you could use a tablespoon of lemon juice and a teaspoon of Splenda instead. Your lamb will be less authentically Caribbean-tasting, but still yummy.

2- to 3-pound section (1–1.5 kilograms) of a leg of lamb

1/2 medium onion, chopped

1/2 teaspoon minced garlic or 1 clove garlic, crushed

1 teaspoon tamarind concentrate

1 tablespoon (15 grams) spicy brown mustard

1 cup (260 grams) canned diced tomatoes

1 teaspoon hot sauce—preferably Caribbean Scotch Bonnet sauce—or more or less to taste

Guar or xanthan (optional)

Place the lamb in your slow cooker.

In a bowl, stir together the onion, garlic, tamarind, mustard, tomatoes, and hot sauce. Pour the mixture over the lamb. Cover the slow cooker, set it to low, and let it cook for a good 8 hours.

When it's done, remove the lamb to a serving platter, thicken the pot juices with the guar or xanthan if it seems necessary, and add salt and pepper to taste.

**YIELD:** 6 servings, each with: 357 calories, 26 g fat, 27 g protein, 3 g carbohydrate, 1 g dietary fiber, 2 g usable carbs.

CHAPTER SEVEN

# Slow Cooker
# Fish and Seafood

I don't generally think of fish when I think of long, slow cooking, and indeed who wants to leave fish in a slow cooker all day? But the gentle, even heating of your slow cooker, used judiciously, can yield fish and seafood that's remarkably moist and tender. When you don't need to have dinner waiting, try these recipes!

Or, as in a few of these recipes, you can cook everything else all day, and then just stir in the seafood for the last little bit of cooking time. It doesn't take long to cook fish or seafood through!

# ⌕ Lime-Basted Scallops

My seafood-loving husband thought these were some of the best scallops he'd ever had.

1/4 cup (60 milliliters) lime juice

3 tablespoons (45 grams) butter

2 cloves garlic

24 ounces (680 grams) sea scallops

Guar or xanthan

1/4 cup (5 grams) chopped fresh cilantro

Put the lime juice, butter, and garlic in your slow cooker. Cover the slow cooker, set it to high, and let it cook for 30 minutes.

Uncover the slow cooker and stir the butter, lime juice, and garlic together. Now add the scallops, stirring them around to coat them with the sauce. Spread them in a single layer on the bottom of the slow cooker. (If the sauce seems to pool in one or two areas, try to cluster the scallops there. In my pot, the sauce liked to stay around the edges.) Re-cover the pot, set it to high, and let it cook for 45 minutes.

When the time's up, remove the scallops to serving plates. Thicken the pot liquid just a tiny bit with guar or xanthan and spoon the sauce over the scallops. Top each serving with a tablespoon of cilantro.

**YIELD:** 4 servings, each with: 233 calories, 10 g fat, 29 g protein, 6 g carbohydrate, trace dietary fiber, 6 g usable carbs.

# ⊡ Lemon-Mustard Salmon Steaks

This is so simple and classic. The salmon comes out tender and moist.

2 tablespoons (28 grams) butter

1 tablespoon (14 milliliters) lemon juice

1 teaspoon Dijon mustard

1 pinch salt or Vege-Sal

2 salmon steaks (totaling about 1 pound/455 grams)

2 tablespoons (8 grams) chopped fresh parsley

Combine the butter, lemon juice, mustard, and salt or Vege-Sal in your slow cooker. Cover the slow cooker, set it to low, and let it cook for 30 to 40 minutes. Stir together.

Now put the salmon steaks in the slow cooker and turn them once or twice to coat. Re-cover the slow cooker and let it cook for 1 hour. Spoon some of the pot liquid over the salmon and sprinkle with the parsley before serving.

**YIELD:** 2 servings, each with: 369 calories, 19 g fat, 46 g protein, 1 g carbohydrate, trace dietary fiber, 1 g usable carbs.

# ⊡ Maple-Balsamic Salmon

This started as a recipe for grilled salmon in *The Low-Carb Barbecue Book*, but it works brilliantly in the slow cooker, as well.

2 salmon steaks (totaling about 1 pound/455 grams)

1 tablespoon (14 milliliters) olive oil

2 tablespoons (60 grams) sugar-free pancake syrup

1 clove garlic, crushed

1 tablespoon (14 milliliters) balsamic vinegar

In your slow cooker, combine everything but the salmon. Cover the slow cooker, set it to low, and let it cook for 30 minutes.

Now add the salmon, turning the steaks to coat them with the sauce. Re-cover the pot and let it cook for 1 hour. Spoon some of the pot liquid over the steaks before serving.

**YIELD:** 2 servings, each with: 326 calories, 15 g fat, 45 g protein, 1 g carbohydrate, trace dietary fiber, 1 g usable carbs.

# Almond-Stuffed Flounder Rolls with Orange Butter Sauce

4 tablespoons (55 grams) butter, divided

2 tablespoons (14 milliliters) lemon juice

1/8 teaspoon orange extract

1 teaspoon Splenda

1/3 cup (145 grams) almonds

1/4 cup (40 grams) minced onion

1 clove garlic, crushed

1 1/2 teaspoons Dijon mustard

1/2 teaspoon soy sauce

1/4 cup (16 grams) minced fresh parsley, divided

1 pound (455 grams) flounder fillets, 4 ounces (115 grams) each

Put 2 tablespoons (28 grams) of the butter, the lemon juice, orange extract, and Splenda in your slow cooker. Cover the slow cooker, set it to low, and let it heat while you fix your flounder rolls.

Put the almonds in a food processor with the S-blade in place and grind them to a cornmeal consistency. Melt 1 tablespoon (14 grams) of butter in a medium-sized heavy skillet and add the ground almonds. Stir the almonds over medium heat for 5 to 7 minutes, or until they smell toasty. Transfer them to a bowl.

Now melt the final tablespoon of butter in the skillet and sauté the onion and garlic over medium-low heat until the onion is just turning translucent. Add them to the almonds and stir them in. Now stir in the mustard, soy sauce, and 2 tablespoons (18 grams) of the parsley.

Lay the flounder fillets on a big plate and divide the almond mixture between them. Spread it over the fillets, and then roll each one up and fasten it with a toothpick.

Take the lid off the slow cooker and stir the sauce. Place the flounder rolls in the sauce and spoon the sauce over them. Re-cover the pot and let the rolls cook for 1 hour. When they're done, spoon the sauce over the rolls and sprinkle the remaining parsley over them to serve.

**YIELD:** 4 servings, each with: 285 calories, 19 g fat, 24 g protein, 5 g carbohydrate, 2 g dietary fiber, 3 g usable carbs.

# Sweet and Sour Shrimp

Adding the shrimp and snow peas at the last moment keeps them from becoming desperately overcooked.

1 cup (220 grams) peaches, peeled and cubed (Frozen unsweetened peaches work well. Just cut them into smaller chunks—1/2 inch.)

1/2 cup (50 grams) chopped onion

1 green bell pepper, diced

1/2 cup (60 grams) chopped celery

1/2 cup (120 milliliters) chicken broth

2 tablespoons (28 milliliters) dark sesame oil

1/4 cup (60 milliliters) soy sauce

2 tablespoons (28 milliliters) rice vinegar

1/4 cup (60 milliliters) lemon juice

1 teaspoon red pepper flakes

1 tablespoon (1.5 grams) Splenda

6 ounces (170 grams) fresh snow pea pods, trimmed

1 1/2 pounds (700 grams) shrimp, shells removed

1/3 cup (95 grams) slivered almonds, toasted

Guar or xanthan

Put the peaches, onion, pepper, celery, broth, sesame oil, soy sauce, vinegar, lemon juice, red pepper flakes, and Splenda in your slow cooker and stir them together. Cover the slow cooker, set it to low, and let it cook for 4 hours. (Or you could cook it on high for 2 hours.)

When the time's up, turn the pot up to high while you trim the snow peas and cut them in 1" lengths. Stir them in and let it cook for 15 to 20 minutes. Now stir in the shrimp. If they're uncooked, give them 10 minutes, or until they're pink through. If they're cooked already, just give them 5 minutes or so, to get hot through.

You can serve this over rice for the carb-eaters in the family, of course. If you like, you can have yours on Cauli-Rice (see recipe page 239), but this dish is high-carb enough already that I'd probably eat it plain.

**YIELD:** 6 servings, each with: 257 calories, 11 g fat, 27 g protein, 13 g carbohydrate, 3 g dietary fiber, 10 g usable carbs.

# Pantry Seafood Supper

This is convenient because, as the name strongly suggests, it uses seafood you've got sitting in your pantry. If, instead, you've got seafood sitting in your freezer, you can use it instead—just let it cook an extra 30 minutes or so to make sure it's thawed and cooked through.

1/4 cup (35 grams) roasted red peppers jarred in oil, diced small (about 1 pepper)

1/3 cup (20 grams) chopped parsley

1 cup (100 grams) chopped mushrooms

3/4 cup (175 milliliters) chicken broth

3/4 cup (175 milliliters) dry white wine

2 tablespoons (20 grams) minced onion

2 teaspoons dried dill weed

1/2 teaspoon paprika

1/2 teaspoon Tabasco sauce

1 cup Carb Countdown dairy beverage

1/4 cup (60 milliliters) heavy cream

Guar or xanthan

6 ounces (170 grams) canned tuna, drained

6 ounces (170 grams) canned crab, drained

6 ounces (170 grams) canned shrimp, drained

Combine the red peppers, parsley, mushrooms, broth, wine, onion, dill, paprika, and Tabasco sauce in your slow cooker. Cover the slow cooker, set it to low, and let it cook for 3 to 4 hours.

When the time's up, stir in the Carb Countdown and cream and thicken the sauce to your liking with guar or xanthan. Now stir in the tuna, crab, and shrimp and let it cook for another 15 to 20 minutes.

Now you have a choice: You can eat this as a chowder, or you can serve it over Cauli-Rice (see recipe page 239) or low-carbohydrate pasta—or even over spaghetti squash. It's up to you.

**YIELD:** 4 servings, each with: 269 calories, 9 g fat, 33 g protein, 4 g carbohydrate, 1 g dietary fiber, 3 g usable carbs.

**CHAPTER EIGHT**

# Slow Cooker
# Crazy Mixed-Up Meals

It's really very hard to organize a cookbook. Take, for instance, the recipes that follow. They really messed up my plan to organize this book largely by protein source. After backing and forthing, moving them around, I threw up my hands and gave them their own chapter.

# ⌂ Simple Meat Loaf

This is simple, but it's hardly boring! Because meat loaf takes at least an hour in the oven, many of you may have given up on it as a weeknight dinner. Baking it in your slow cooker works remarkably well, although it doesn't brown much.

1 pound (455 grams) ground round

1 pound (455 grams) pork sausage

1 medium onion, finely chopped

1 medium green pepper, finely chopped

1/4 cup (25 grams) oat bran

1/2 teaspoon pepper

1/2 teaspoon salt or Vege-Sal

2 tablespoons (30 grams) Worcestershire sauce

2 eggs

1/2 cup (60 grams) pork rind crumbs (Run pork rinds through your food processor or blender.)

Place all ingredients in a big mixing bowl and use clean hands to smoosh everything together until it's well blended.

Put a rack or a collapsible basket-style steamer in the bottom of your slow cooker. Fold two squares of foil into strips and criss-cross them on the rack or steamer and up the sides of the slow cooker. (What you're doing is making a sling to help you lift the loaf out of the slow cooker.) If the holes/slots in your rack are pretty big, put a sheet of foil over the criss-crossed strips and pierce it all over with a fork.

Place the meat mixture on top of this and form into an evenly-domed meat loaf, smoothing the surface with dampened hands. Cover the slow cooker, set it to low, and let it cook for 9 to 12 hours.

Use the foil strips to lift the meat loaf out of the slow cooker.

**YIELD:** 8 servings, each with: 438 calories, 36 g fat, 23 g protein, 6 g carbohydrate, 1 g dietary fiber, 5 g usable carbs.

# Morty's Mixed Meat Loaf

The combination of meats makes this loaf unusually tasty.

2 slices cooked bacon, crumbled

1 pound (455 grams) ground round

1 pound (455 grams) ground pork

1 pound (455 grams) ground turkey

3 stalks celery, finely chopped

1/2 cup (30 grams) finely chopped fresh parsley

1/2 cup (120 grams) Dana's No-Sugar Ketchup (see recipe page 228)
   or purchased low-carb ketchup

1 teaspoon hot sauce

2 eggs

1/2 cup (60 grams) barbecue-style pork rind crumbs
   (Just run 'em through your food processor.)

2 tablespoons (28 ml) Worcestershire sauce

1 teaspoon lemon juice

1/2 teaspoon dried marjoram

1 teaspoon salt or Vege-Sal

1/2 teaspoon pepper

Put a rack or basket-style steamer in the bottom of your slow cooker pot. Fold two squares of foil into strips and criss-cross them on the rack or steamer and up the sides of the slow cooker. (What you're doing is making a sling to help you lift the loaf out of the slow cooker.) If the holes/slots in your rack are pretty big, put a sheet of foil over the criss-crossed strips and pierce it all over with a fork.

Place all your ingredients in a big bowl and, using clean hands, smoosh everything together really well. Form it into a round loaf on the rack in the slow cooker. Cover the slow cooker, set it to low, and let it cook for 8 to 10 hours.

Use the strips of foil to lift the loaf out of the slow cooker.

**YIELD:** 8 servings, each with: 453 calories, 30 g fat, 37 g protein, 7 g carbohydrate, 2 g dietary fiber, 5 g usable carbs.

# Pizza Stew

Here's a slow cooker meal for your pizza-craving family. Maria gets the credit for perfecting this one. It wasn't quite right the way I originally conceived it. Maria gave me feedback, we went with her suggestions, and success was ours!

> 1 pound (455 grams) bulk Italian sausage
>
> 1 pound (455 grams) ground round
>
> 1 green bell pepper, diced
>
> 1/4 cup (25 grams) diced onion
>
> 14 ounces (425 milliliters) no-sugar-added pizza sauce (Ragu makes one.)
>
> 2 cups (220 grams) shredded mozzarella cheese
>
> 1/2 cup (40 grams) shredded Parmesan cheese

In a big, heavy skillet, brown and crumble the sausage and beef together. Drain them well and transfer them to your slow cooker. Add the pepper and onion and stir. Stir in the pizza sauce. Cover the slow cooker, set it to low, and let it cook for 5 to 6 hours.

Now uncover the slow cooker and top the stew with the mozzarella cheese. Re-cover the slow cooker and let it cook for another 30 to 45 minutes, to melt the cheese. Serve with the Parmesan cheese sprinkled on top.

**YIELD:** 6 servings, each with: 626 calories, 49 g fat, 37 g protein, 8 g carbohydrate, 2 g dietary fiber, 6 g usable carbs.

# 🍲 Low-Carb Slow Cooker Paella

Maria, who tested this, rates it a 10. She added, "While this won't fool a purist, the flavor is quite good. For those who can't afford saffron, turmeric is an acceptable substitute. For an authentic presentation, which is important, put the 'rice' in a paella pan or flat casserole, mix it with the veggies, and arrange the chicken and shrimp artistically on top." Do look for Spanish chorizo, rather than Mexican chorizo, for this dish.

6 chicken leg and side quarters (about 3 pounds/1.5 kilograms)
1/4 cup (60 milliliters) olive oil
1 cup (130 grams) chopped onion
1 clove garlic, crushed
1 green bell pepper
6 ounces (170 grams) chorizo links or diced ham
14 1/2 ounces (411 grams) canned tomato wedges, drained
1/2 teaspoon saffron threads
1 cup (235 milliliters) chicken broth
1 teaspoon chicken bouillon concentrate
6 ounces (170 grams) shrimp
1/2 cup (40 grams) fresh snow pea pods, cut into 1/2" pieces
1 head cauliflower

In a big, heavy skillet, brown the chicken in the oil.

While that's happening, put the onion, garlic, and green pepper in your slow cooker. When the chicken is brown, transfer it to the slow cooker as well.

If using chorizo, slice it into rounds and brown it in the same skillet, then transfer it to the slow cooker. If using ham, you can simply add it directly to the slow cooker. Place the tomatoes on top of that.

In a bowl, mix together the saffron, broth, and bouillon and pour it into the slow cooker. Cover the slow cooker, set it to low, and let it cook for 6 hours.

When the time's up, turn the slow cooker to high. Add the shrimp and snow peas to the slow cooker, re-cover, and cook for another 30 minutes.

While that's happening, shred the cauliflower in your food processor, put it in a microwavable casserole dish with a lid, add a few tablespoons of water, cover, and microwave it on high for 8 to 9 minutes. Serve with the paella.

**YIELD:** 8 servings, each with: 599 calories, 42 g fat, 46 g protein, 8 g carbohydrate, 1 g dietary fiber, 7 g usable carbs.

# Albondigas en Salsa Chipotle

Mexican meatballs! Yummy.

1/2 medium onion, chopped

1 tablespoon (14 milliliters) oil

1 teaspoon ground cumin

1 teaspoon ground coriander

3 cloves garlic, crushed

1 teaspoon dried oregano

1 teaspoon dried thyme

14 1/2 ounces (411 grams) canned tomatoes with green chiles, drained

1 cup (235 milliliters) chicken broth

1/2 teaspoon chicken bouillon concentrate

1 chipotle chile canned in adobo sauce, or more to taste

1 pound (455 grams) ground round

1 pound (455 grams) ground turkey

1 egg

1 teaspoon pepper

1/2 teaspoon ground allspice

1/2 teaspoon ground cumin

1/2 teaspoon ground coriander

1 teaspoon dried oregano

2 teaspoons salt or Vege-Sal

1/2 medium onion, finely chopped

3 cloves garlic, crushed

2 tablespoons (28 milliliters) olive oil

1 teaspoon guar or xanthan

In a big, heavy skillet, sauté 1/2 onion in the 1 tablespoon oil over medium-high heat until translucent. Add the 1 teaspoon ground cumin, 1 teaspoon ground coriander, 3 cloves garlic, 1 teaspoon oregano, and 1 teaspoon thyme and sauté for another minute or two. Transfer the mixture to your blender or food processor.

Add the tomatoes, broth, bouillon, and chipotle. Blend until smooth and pour into your slow cooker. Cover the slow cooker, set it to low, and start it cooking as you make the meatballs.

Place the beef, turkey, egg, pepper, allspice, 1/2 teaspoon ground cumin, 1/2 teaspoon ground coriander, 1 teaspoon oregano, salt or Vege-Sal, 1/2 onion, and 3 cloves garlic into a big bowl and use clean hands to smoosh it all together. Form it into meatballs.

In the skillet, heat 2 tablespoons oil over medium-high heat and brown the meatballs on all sides. Transfer the meatballs to the slow cooker, re-cover, and let the whole thing cook for 3 to 4 hours.

Scoop the meatballs out with a slotted spoon and put them in a serving bowl. Thicken the sauce to taste with the guar or xanthan and pour the sauce over the meatballs.

**YIELD:** 8 servings, each with: 297 calories, 20 g fat, 23 g protein, 5 g carbohydrate, 1 g dietary fiber, 4 g usable carbs.

# Brunswick Stew

This is an old favorite, decarbed and updated for your slow cooker.

> 1 large onion, sliced
> 2 pounds (1 kilogram) skinless chicken thighs
> 1 1/2 cups (210 grams) ham cubes, cooked
> 1 teaspoon dry mustard
> 1 teaspoon dried thyme
> 1/2 teaspoon pepper
> 1 cup (260 grams) canned diced tomatoes
> 14 ounces (400 grams) chicken broth
> 3 cloves garlic, crushed
> 1 tablespoon (16 grams) Worcestershire sauce
> 1/4 teaspoon hot sauce, or to taste
> 1 cup (170 grams) canned black soybeans, drained

Place the onion in your slow cooker first. Add the chicken and ham.

In a bowl, mix together the dry mustard, thyme, pepper, tomatoes, broth, garlic, Worcestershire sauce, and hot sauce. Pour the mixture over the chicken and ham. Cover the slow cooker, set it to low, and let it cook for 8 hours.

When the time's up, stir in the soybeans and let the whole thing cook for another 20 minutes or so.

**YIELD:** 6 servings, each with: 212 calories, 10 g fat, 21 g protein, 9 g carbohydrate, 3 g dietary fiber, 6 g usable carbs.

CHAPTER NINE

# Slow Cooker Soups

If there's a type of dish for which the slow cooker seems custom-made, it's soups. How wonderful to come home tired on a cold evening to a pot of hot, hearty, homemade soup!

# Black Bean Soup

One of the few carb-y dishes I sometimes miss is legume soup, especially black bean soup. This is my decarbed version.

28 ounces (800 grams) canned black soybeans

14 ounces (400 grams) canned black beans

2 cups (475 milliliters) chicken broth

1 medium onion, cut into chunks

4 cloves garlic, crushed

1 medium carrot, shredded

2 medium stalks celery, finely diced

1 teaspoon salt or Vege-Sal

1/2 teaspoon pepper

1 tablespoon (14 milliliters) liquid smoke flavoring

2 teaspoons hot sauce

2 cups (230 grams) ham cubes

Using your food processor with the S-blade in place, puree the soybeans and black beans. Place them in your slow cooker. Stir in the broth.

Place the onion in the food processor. Add the garlic, carrot, and celery. Pulse the food processor until everything is finely chopped. Add to the soup.

Stir in the salt or Vege-Sal, pepper, liquid smoke flavoring, hot sauce, and ham. Cover the slow cooker, set it to low, and let it cook for 9 to 10 hours.

When the time's up, stir the soup up (it'll have settled out some) and check to see if it needs more salt and pepper. (This will depend on how salty your ham is.)

YIELD: 8 servings, each with: 218 calories, 9 g fat, 19 g protein, 17 g carbohydrate, 9 g dietary fiber, 8 g usable carbs.

# ⛯ Bollito Misto

All this Italian soup-stew needs with it is a green salad, and maybe some crusty bread for the carb-eaters.

1 large onion, sliced

2 carrots, cut 1/2" thick

3 stalks celery, cut 1/2" thick

2 pounds (1 kilogram) beef round, cubed

1/2 teaspoon salt

1/2 teaspoon pepper

2 tablespoons (8 grams) chopped fresh parsley

1 bay leaf

3 teaspoons chicken bouillon concentrate

1 quart (9400 milliliters) chicken broth

2 pounds (1 kilogram) boneless, skinless chicken thighs, cubed

1 pound (455 grams) Italian sausage links

1/2 cup (130 grams) purchased pesto sauce

Put the onion, carrots, and celery in your slow cooker. Season the beef with the salt and pepper and place them on top. Add the parsley and bay leaf. Stir the bouillon into the chicken and pour it into the slow cooker. Cover the slow cooker, set it to low, and let it cook for 5 to 6 hours.

Add the chicken, turn the heat up to high, and let the whole thing cook another hour.

While it's cooking, pour yourself a glass of Chianti, and put out some vegetables and dip for the kids. In a big, heavy skillet, place the sausages, cover with water, slap a lid on, and simmer for 20 minutes over medium heat. Remove the skillet from the heat and leave the sausages in the water, with the lid on.

When the slow cooker's time is up, drain the sausage and cut it into 1" chunks. Stir the sausage into the stuff in the slow cooker. Now ladle the whole thing into soup bowls and top each serving with a tablespoon of pesto.

**YIELD:** 8 servings, each with: 599 calories, 43 g fat, 44 g protein, 6 g carbohydrate, 1 g dietary fiber, 5 g usable carbs.

# Cauliflower, Cheese, and Spinach Soup

Maria's family gave this raves. It's easy, too!

6 cups (900 grams) cauliflower florets, cut into 1/2" pieces

1 quart (9400 milliliters) chicken broth

1/2 cup (80 grams) minced red onion

5 ounces (140 grams) bagged baby spinach leaves, pre-washed

1/4 teaspoon cayenne

1/2 teaspoon salt or Vege-Sal

1/4 teaspoon pepper

4 cloves garlic, crushed

3 cups (675 grams) shredded smoked Gouda cheese

1 cup (235 milliliters) Carb Countdown dairy beverage

Guar or xanthan

In your slow cooker, combine the cauliflower, broth, onion, spinach, cayenne, salt or Vege-Sal, pepper, and garlic. Cover the slow cooker, set it to low, and let it cook for 6 hours, or until the cauliflower is tender.

When the time's up, stir in the Gouda, a little at a time, and then the Carb Countdown. Re-cover the slow cooker and cook for another 15 minutes, or until the cheese has thoroughly melted. Thicken soup a little with guar or xanthan.

YIELD: 8 servings, each with: 214 calories, 14 g fat, 17 g protein, 7 g carbohydrate, 2 g dietary fiber, 5 g usable carbs.

# ⟨ᴉ⟩ Cream of UnPotato Soup

I never cease to marvel at the versatility of cauliflower. This really does taste like potato soup.

> 1 quart (9400 milliliters) chicken broth
> 1/2 head cauliflower, chunked
> 1/2 cup (50 grams) chopped onion
> 1/2 cup (50 grams) Ketatoes mix
> 1/2 cup (120 milliliters) heavy cream
> 1/2 cup (120 milliliters) Carb Countdown dairy beverage
> Guar or xanthan (optional)
> 5 scallions, sliced

Put the broth, cauliflower, and onion in your slow cooker. Cover the slow cooker, set it to low, and let it cook for 4 to 5 hours.

I use a hand blender to puree my soup right in the slow cooker, but you may transfer the cauliflower and onion, along with a cup of broth, into your blender or food processor instead. Either way, puree until completely smooth, then blend in the Ketatoes. If you have removed the cauliflower from the slow cooker to puree, pour the puree back in, and whisk it into the remaining broth.

Stir in the cream and Carb Countdown. Thicken it a bit further with guar or xanthan if you feel it needs it. Add salt and pepper to taste and stir in the sliced scallions. Serve hot right away or chill and serve as vichyssoise.

**YIELD:** 6 servings, each with: 190 calories, 11 g fat, 12 g protein, 13 g carbohydrate, 6 g dietary fiber, 7 g usable carbs.

#  German UnPotato Soup

This is worth the time you spend cutting things up! It's hearty and filling.

1 head cauliflower, chunked

2 stalks celery, sliced

1 medium onion, chopped

8 ounces (225 grams) smoked sausage, sliced

1 tablespoon (28 milliliters) oil

4 cups (950 milliliters) beef broth

2 tablespoons (28 milliliters) vinegar

1 tablespoon (1.5 grams) Splenda

1/4 teaspoon celery seed

1/2 teaspoon dry mustard

1/4 teaspoon pepper

2 cups (240 grams) bagged coleslaw mix

Place the cauliflower, celery, and onion in your slow cooker.

In a big, heavy skillet, brown the sausage a bit in the oil. Transfer the sausage to the slow cooker, too.

Pour 1 cup of the broth into the skillet and stir it around a bit to dissolve the flavorful bits. Pour it into the slow cooker.

In a bowl, combine the rest of the broth with the vinegar, Splenda, celery seed, dry mustard, and pepper. Pour over the vegetables and sausage. Cover the slow cooker, set it to low, and let it cook for 8 hours.

When the time's up, stir in the coleslaw mix and let it cook for another 20 to 30 minutes.

**YIELD:** 4 servings, each with: 344 calories, 22 g fat, 20 g protein, 17 g carbohydrate, 2 g dietary fiber, 15 g usable carbs.

# Maria's New England Clam Chowder

This one is from my tester and dear friend Maria. She says, "This was so good that I called my brother Peter over and made him try it. He was very impressed. He's a big clam chowder fan, and he said that our grandmother would approve."

4 slices bacon, diced

1 medium onion, chopped

1 large turnip, cut in 1/2" cubes

16 ounces (455 grams) canned clams, undrained

3 cloves garlic, crushed

1 teaspoon salt

1/2 teaspoon pepper

2 cups (475 milliliters) heavy cream

2 tablespoons (28 grams) butter

In a big, heavy skillet, sauté the bacon, onion, and turnip until the onion is golden. Drain and put it on the bottom of your slow cooker.

Pour the clam liquid into a 2-cup measuring cup and add enough water to make 2 cups. In a bowl, combine the liquid and water mixture, the clams, garlic, salt, and pepper. Pour the mixture into the slow cooker. Cover the slow cooker, set it to low, and let it cook for 5 hours, or until the turnips are tender. Blend in the cream and butter during the last 45 minutes of cooking.

**YIELD:** 5 servings, each with: 550 calories, 44 g fat, 27 g protein, 11 g carbohydrate, 1 g dietary fiber, 10 g usable carbs.

# Cream of Mushroom Soup

If you've only ever thought of mushroom soup as gooey stuff that came in cans and was used in casseroles, you need to try this! It has a rich, earthy flavor. Even my mushroom-phobic husband liked it.

8 ounces (225 grams) mushrooms, sliced

1/4 cup (25 grams) chopped onion

2 tablespoons (28 grams) butter

1 quart (9400 milliliters) chicken broth

1/2 cup (120 milliliters) heavy cream

1/2 cup (120 grams) light sour cream

Guar or xanthan (optional)

In a big, heavy skillet, sauté the mushrooms and onion in the butter until the mushrooms soften and change color. Transfer them to your slow cooker. Add the broth. Cover the slow cooker, set it to low, and let it cook for 5 to 6 hours.

When the time's up, scoop out the vegetables with a slotted spoon and put them in your blender or food processor. Add enough broth to help them process easily and puree them finely. Pour the pureed vegetables back into the slow cooker, scraping out every last bit with a rubber scraper. Now stir in the heavy cream and sour cream and add salt and pepper to taste. Thicken the sauce a bit with guar or xanthan if you think it needs it. Serve immediately.

YIELD: 5 servings, each with: 176 calories, 15 g fat, 6 g protein, 5 g carbohydrate, 1 g dietary fiber, 4 usable carbs.

# Chicken and Vegetable Soup with Thai Spices

This soup is light, fragrant, and wonderful.

2 tablespoons (28 milliliters) oil

2 carrots, thinly sliced

4 stalks celery, thinly sliced

2 cups (200 grams) sliced mushrooms

1/2 medium onion, thinly sliced

2 cloves garlic, crushed

1 1/2 pounds (700 grams) boneless, skinless chicken breast, cut into 1/2" cubes

2 quarts (2 liters) chicken broth

2 cups (300 grams) frozen cross-cut green beans

1 tablespoon (8 grams) grated ginger root

9 teaspoons chili paste

1 tablespoon (14 milliliters) lemon juice

1 tablespoon (14 milliliters) lime juice

1/8 teaspoon anise seed, ground

1/4 teaspoon ground cardamom

1/4 teaspoon ground cinnamon

1/2 teaspoon ground cumin

1/4 teaspoon ground coriander

1 tablespoon (18 grams) fish sauce

Fresh cilantro

Heat the oil in a big, heavy skillet over medium-high heat and sauté the carrots, celery, mushrooms, and onion until the onion is starting to get translucent. Transfer them to your slow cooker, adding the garlic. Now add the chicken to the skillet and sauté just until it's sealed on the outside. Transfer it to the slow cooker, too.

Pour in the broth and add the green beans, ginger, chili paste, lemon juice, lime juice, anise seed, cardamom, cinnamon, cumin, coriander, and fish sauce. Stir, cover the slow cooker, set it to low, and let it cook for 6 to 8 hours.

Scatter a little cilantro over each bowlful before serving.

**YIELD:** 8 servings, each with: 209 calories, 8 g fat, 25 g protein, 9 g carbohydrate, 2 g dietary fiber, 7 g usable carbs.

# Chicken Soup with Wild Rice

Wild rice has more fiber, and therefore fewer usable carbs, than regular rice, either white or brown. And it adds a certain cachet to your soup!

2 quarts (2 liters) chicken broth

2 carrots, thinly sliced

2 stalks celery, diced

1/2 cup (50 grams) chopped onion

1 pound (455 grams) boneless, skinless chicken breast, cut into 1/2" cubes

1/4 cup (40 grams) wild rice

1 teaspoon poultry seasoning

Simply combine everything in your slow cooker, cover, set it to low, and let it cook for 6 to 7 hours.

**YIELD:** 6 servings, each with: 182 calories, 4 g fat, 25 g protein, 10 g carbohydrate, 2 g dietary fiber, 8 g usable carbs.

# Mexican Beef and Bean Soup

You know the family will love this!

12 ounces (340 grams) ground round

1 medium onion, chopped

2 cloves garlic, crushed

1 medium green bell pepper, diced

1 quart (9400 milliliters) beef broth

1 teaspoon beef bouillon concentrate

14 1/2 ounces (411 grams) canned tomatoes with green chiles

15 ounces (425 grams) canned black soybeans

2 teaspoons ground coriander

1 teaspoon ground cumin

4 tablespoons (16 grams) chopped cilantro

6 tablespoons (70 grams) sour cream

In a big, heavy skillet, brown and crumble the ground beef. Drain it well and transfer it to your slow cooker.

Add the onion, garlic, bell pepper, broth, bouillon, tomatoes, soybeans, coriander, and cumin and stir. Cover the slow cooker, set it to low, and let it cook for 7 to 8 hours.

Top each bowlful with cilantro and sour cream.

**YIELD:** 6 servings, each with: 296 calories, 16 g fat, 25 g protein, 14 g carbohydrate, 5 g dietary fiber, 9 g usable carbs.

# Chicken Minestrone

Here's a decarbed version of the Italian favorite. You'll never miss the pasta!

3 slices bacon, chopped

1 medium onion, chopped

2 medium turnips, cut into $1/2$" cubes

1 medium carrot, thinly sliced

2 small zucchini, quartered and sliced

2 stalks celery, thinly sliced

3 tablespoons (45 milliliters) olive oil

1 $1/2$ quarts (1.5 liters) chicken broth

1 $1/2$ pounds (700 grams) skinless chicken thighs, boned and cubed

1 tablespoon (4 grams) Italian seasoning

14 $1/2$ ounces (411 grams) canned diced tomatoes, undrained

15 ounces (425 grams) canned black soybeans

Spray a big, heavy skillet with nonstick cooking spray, then start the bacon frying over medium heat. As some grease cooks out of the bacon, add as many of the vegetables as will fit and sauté them until they soften just a bit. Transfer the vegetables to your slow cooker and continue sautéing the rest of the vegetables, adding oil as needed, until all the vegetables are softened a bit, and in the slow cooker.

Place the broth, chicken, Italian seasoning, tomatoes, soybeans, and salt and pepper to taste in the slow cooker. Cover the slow cooker, set it to low, and let it cook for 7 to 8 hours.

**YIELD:** 6 servings, each with: 294 calories, 16 g fat, 21 g protein, 18 g carbohydrate, 6 g dietary fiber, 12 g usable carbs.

# Spicy Chicken and Mushroom Soup

This is exotic and delicious.

3 tablespoons (45 grams) butter

1 leek, thinly sliced (white part only)

8 ounces (225 grams) sliced mushrooms

1 clove garlic, crushed

2 teaspoons Garam Masala (see recipe page 236) or purchased garam masala

1 teaspoon pepper

1/4 teaspoon cayenne

1/4 teaspoon ground nutmeg

1 quart (9400 milliliters) chicken broth

12 ounces (340 grams) boneless, skinless chicken breasts, cut into thin strips

1/2 cup (120 milliliters) Carb Countdown dairy beverage

1/2 cup (120 milliliters) heavy cream

3 tablespoons (12 grams) chopped fresh cilantro (optional)

Melt the butter in a big, heavy skillet, over medium heat, and sauté the leek with the mushrooms until they both soften. Stir in the garlic, Garam Masala, pepper, cayenne, and nutmeg and sauté for another minute or two. Transfer to your slow cooker. Pour in the broth and add the chicken. Cover the slow cooker, set it to low, and let it cook for 6 to 7 hours.

When the time's up, use a slotted spoon to scoop roughly two-thirds of the solids into your blender or food processor. Add a cup or so of the broth and puree until smooth. Stir the puree back into the rest of the soup. (You may want to rinse the blender or food processor out with a little broth, to get all of the puree.) Stir in the Carb Countdown and cream. Re-cover the pot and let it cook for another 30 minutes. Serve with cilantro on top. Or not, if you prefer, it's nice without it, too!

**YIELD:** 6 servings, each with: 243 calories, 16 g fat, 18 g protein, 6 g carbohydrate, 1 g dietary fiber, 5 g usable carbs.

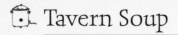 Tavern Soup

Cheese soup with beer! Don't worry about the kids, the alcohol cooks off.

    1 1/2 quarts (1.5 liters) chicken broth
    1/4 cup (30 grams) finely diced celery
    1/4 cup (30 grams) finely diced green bell pepper
    1/4 cup (30 grams) shredded carrot
    1/4 cup (16 grams) chopped fresh parsley
    1/2 teaspoon pepper
    1 pound (455 grams) sharp cheddar cheese, shredded
    12 ounces (355 milliliters) light beer
    1/2 teaspoon salt or Vege-Sal
    1/4 teaspoon Tabasco sauce
    Guar or xanthan

Combine the broth, celery, green pepper, carrot, parsley, and pepper in your slow cooker. Cover the slow cooker, set it to low, and let it cook for 6 to 8 hours, and even a bit longer won't hurt.

When the time's up, either use a hand-held blender to puree the vegetables right there in the slow cooker or scoop them out with a slotted spoon, puree them in your blender, and return them to the slow cooker.

Now whisk in the cheese a little at a time, until it's all melted in. Add the beer, salt or Vege-Sal, and Tabasco sauce and stir till the foaming stops. Use guar or xanthan to thicken your soup until it's about the texture of heavy cream. Re-cover the pot, turn it to high, and let it cook for another 20 minutes before serving.

**YIELD:** 8 servings, each with: 274 calories, 20 g fat, 18 g protein, 3 g carbohydrate, trace dietary fiber, 3 g usable carbs.

# Turkey Sausage Soup

This is a great, filling family soup for a cold night.

1 1/2 pounds (700 grams) bulk turkey sausage

14 1/2 ounces (411 grams) canned diced tomatoes

8 ounces (225 grams) canned, sliced mushrooms

1 turnip, diced

1 cup (150 grams) cauliflower, diced

1/2 cup (50 grams) chopped onion

1 cup (120 grams) chopped green bell pepper

1 quart (9400 milliliters) chicken broth

2 teaspoons chicken bouillon concentrate

1 teaspoon dried basil

2 teaspoons prepared horseradish

1 cup (235 milliliters) heavy cream

In a large, heavy skillet, brown and crumble the sausage. Pour off the fat and put the sausage in your slow cooker. Add the tomatoes, mushrooms, turnip, cauliflower, onion, and green pepper.

In a bowl, stir the broth and bouillon together. Stir in the basil and horseradish. Pour the mixture into the slow cooker. Cover the slow cooker, set it to low, and let it cook for 7 to 8 hours.

When the time's up, stir in the cream and let it cook for another 10 to 15 minutes.

**YIELD:** 6 servings, each with: 666 calories, 61 g fat, 17 g protein, 12 g carbohydrate, 2 g dietary fiber, 10 g usable carbs.

# Seafood Chowder

My sister Kim, who tested this for me, said that you don't have to stick to shrimp. You could use crab, chunks of lobster tail, or even a cut-up firm-fleshed fish fillet. Don't use fake seafood—"delicacies" and such. It has a lot of added carbs.

1 1/2 cups (225 grams) shredded cauliflower

1/3 cup (40 grams) shredded carrots

1 teaspoon dried thyme

1 clove garlic

1 tablespoon (10 grams) finely minced green bell pepper

1/8 teaspoon cayenne

1/4 teaspoon pepper

3 cups (700 milliliters) chicken broth

1 cup (235 milliliters) Carb Countdown dairy beverage

1/4 cup (60 milliliters) heavy cream

8 ounces (225 grams) shrimp, shells removed

1 tablespoon (5 grams) Ketatoes mix

1/4 cup (25 grams) scallions, thinly sliced

Guar or xanthan

Combine the cauliflower, carrots, thyme, garlic, green pepper, cayenne, pepper, and broth in your slow cooker. Cover the slow cooker, set it to low, and let it cook for 4 hours.

Turn the slow cooker to high and stir in the Carb Countdown and cream. Re-cover the slow cooker and let it cook for another 30 to 45 minutes. If your shrimp are big, chop them coarsely during this time, but little, whole shrimp will look prettier, of course!

Stir in the Ketotoes mix. Now stir in the shrimp and re-cover the pot. If your shrimp are pre-cooked, just give them 5 minutes or so to heat through. If they're raw, give them 10 minutes. Stir in the scallions and salt to taste. Thicken the broth with the guar or xanthan.

**YIELD:** 5 servings, each with: 164 calories, 8 g fat, 17 g protein, 7 g carbohydrate, 2 g dietary fiber, 5 g usable carbs.

# CHAPTER TEN

# Slow Cooker Sides

My guess is you use your slow cooker mostly for main dishes, because that's the way it'll make your life the most convenient. Many of the main dishes in this book are complete meals, full of vegetables as well as protein, and they don't need a thing with them except a beverage. With the main dishes that do need a side, the easiest and most appealing thing is often a salad.

Yet there are good reasons to cook a side dish in your slow cooker. Some of them just plain take less work and watching this way, like the Southern Beans. Sometimes you want to make an interesting side to go with a plain meat roasting in the oven and want to be able to ignore it for an hour or two or three while you do something else. In both of these instances, the slow cooker is your very good friend.

# Barbecue Green Beans

These are fab!

> 4 cups (600 grams) cross-cut frozen green beans, unthawed
>
> 1/4 cup (25 grams) chopped onion
>
> 4 slices cooked bacon, drained and crumbled
>
> 1/3 cup (75 milliliters) low-carb barbecue sauce
> (see recipe page 231 or use purchased sauce)

Put the green beans in your slow cooker. Add the onion and bacon, then stir in the barbecue sauce. Cover the slow cooker, set it to high, and let it cook for 3 hours. (If you prefer, set it to low and let it cook for 5 to 6 hours.)

**YIELD:** 6 servings, each with: 58 calories, 2 g fat, 3 g protein, 8 g carbohydrate, 2 g dietary fiber, 6 g usable carbs.

# Southern Beans

Southerners will be shocked to know that I never tasted green beans slowly cooked with bacon until I moved to southern Indiana, but I liked them right off. Around our house, this recipe is jokingly referred to as The Sacred Masonic Vegetable, because my husband's never been to a Masonic banquet that didn't feature beans cooked this way!

> 4 cups (600 grams) frozen green beans, unthawed
>
> 1/3 cup (35 grams) diced onion
>
> 1/4 cup (30 grams) diced celery
>
> 4 slices bacon, cooked and crumbled
>
> 1 tablespoon (18 milliliters) bacon grease
>
> 1/2 cup (120 milliliters) water

Place the beans in the slow cooker and stir in everything else. Cover the slow cooker, set it to low, and let it cook for 4 hours.

**YIELD:** 6 servings, each with: 75 calories, 4 g fat, 3 g protein, 7 g carbohydrate, 3 g dietary fiber, 4 g usable carbs.

## Tangy Beans

4 cups (600 grams) frozen green beans, unthawed

1/4 cup (25 grams) chopped onion

1/4 cup (30 grams) chopped green bell pepper

1/4 cup (60 milliliters) cider vinegar

2 tablespoons (3 grams) Splenda

1/8 teaspoon black pepper

Combine everything in your slow cooker. Stir to distribute evenly. Cover the slow cooker, set it to low, and let it cook for 5 hours.

Serve with a pat of butter and a little salt.

**YIELD:** 4 servings, each with: 50 calories, trace fat, 2 g protein, 12 g carbohydrate, 4 g dietary fiber, 8 g usable carbs.

# Green Bean Casserole

28 ounces (800 grams) frozen green beans, unthawed

1 cup (100 grams) chopped mushrooms

1/4 cup (35 grams) roasted red pepper, diced

1/4 cup (25 grams) chopped onion

2 teaspoons dried sage

1 teaspoon salt or Vege-Sal

1 teaspoon pepper

1/2 teaspoon ground nutmeg

1 cup (235 milliliters) beef broth

1 teaspoon beef bouillon concentrate

1/2 cup (120 milliliters) heavy cream

Guar or xanthan

3/4 cup (95 grams) slivered almonds

1 tablespoon (14 grams) butter

Combine the green beans, mushrooms, red pepper, and onion in your slow cooker.

In a bowl, mix together the sage, salt or Vege-Sal, pepper, nutmeg, broth, and bouillon. Pour the mixture over the vegetables. Stir the whole thing up. Cover the slow cooker, set it to low, and let it cook for 5 to 6 hours.

When the time's up, stir in the cream and thicken the sauce a bit with guar or xanthan. Re-cover the slow cooker and let it stay hot while you sauté the almonds in the butter until golden. Stir them into the beans.

**YIELD:** 8 servings, each with: 191 calories, 14 g fat, 7 g protein, 12 g carbohydrate, 4 g dietary fiber, 8 g usable carbs.

# Basic Artichokes

2 artichokes
1/4 cup (60 milliliters) lemon juice

Using kitchen shears, snip the pointy tips off the artichoke leaves. Split the artichokes down the middle, top to bottom, and scrape out the chokes.

Fill your slow cooker with water, add the lemon juice, and put in the artichokes. Cover the slow cooker, set it to high, and let it cook for 3 to 4 hours.

Drain the artichokes.

Serve the artichokes with the dipping sauce of your choice, such as lemon butter, mayonnaise, aioli, chipotle mayonnaise, whatever you've got. If you have a big slow cooker, feel free to cook more artichokes!

**YIELD:** 2 servings, each with: 68 calories, trace fat, 4 g protein, 16 g carbohydrate, 7 g dietary fiber, 9 g usable carbs.


# Maria's Slow Cooker Asparagus

Here's another recipe contributed by my pal and recipe tester Maria.

1 pound (455 grams) asparagus spears
1 teaspoon dried rosemary
1 clove garlic, crushed
1 tablespoon (28 milliliters) lemon juice

Cut off woody ends of the asparagus. Place trimmed asparagus on the bottom of your slow cooker. (If you're using a round cooker, you may need to cut them to fit.) Sprinkle the asparagus with the rosemary and garlic and pour the lemon juice on top. Cover the slow cooker, set it to low, and let it cook for 2 hours, or until the asparagus is tender.

**YIELD:** 4 servings, each with: 17 calories, trace fat, 1 g protein, 4 g carbohydrate, 1 g dietary fiber, 3 g usable carbs.

# Spinach Parmesan Casserole

This is a lot like creamed spinach, only less—well, creamy.

20 ounces (570 grams) frozen chopped spinach, thawed and drained*

1/3 cup (75 milliliters) heavy cream

1/2 cup (40 grams) shredded Parmesan cheese

1 clove garlic, crushed

2 tablespoons (20 grams) minced onion

1 egg

1/2 teaspoon salt

Place all ingredients in a mixing bowl. Stir it to blend very well. Spray a 6-cup glass casserole dish with nonstick cooking spray. Put the spinach mixture in the casserole, smoothing the top.

Place the casserole dish in your slow cooker and carefully pour water around it up to 1" of the rim. Cover the slow cooker, set it to low, and let it cook for 4 hours.

Uncover the slow cooker and turn it off at least 30 minutes before serving time, so the water cools enough that you can remove the dish without scalding yourself.

*Make sure your spinach is very well drained. It's best to put it in a colander and press it as hard as you can, turning it several times.

YIELD: 6 servings, each with: 109 calories, 8 g fat, 7 g protein, 5 g carbohydrate, 3 g dietary fiber, 2 g usable carbs.

# Macadangdang

Long-time readers know that I'm a big fan of Peg Bracken and her cookbooks. This is my decarbed version of Macadangdang Spinach Medley, which appeared in Peg's *I Hate To Cook Almanac*. It's named for her Aunt Henry Macadangdang, who married a Filipino gentleman of that name. I found the name so charming and euphonious, I thought I'd just call this version Macadangdang. My husband rates this a perfect 10, and I like it, too!

1/2 head cauliflower

10 ounces (280 grams) frozen chopped spinach, thawed and drained

2 tablespoons (28 grams) butter

1/2 cup (25 grams) chopped onion

1 clove garlic, crushed

4 eggs

1/2 cup (120 milliliters) Carb Countdown dairy beverage

1 1/2 teaspoons salt or Vege-Sal

1/4 teaspoon pepper

1/2 cup (40 grams) grated Parmesan cheese

1 cup (110 grams) shredded mozzarella cheese

Run the cauliflower through the shredding blade of your food processor. Place the resulting Cauli-Rice in a mixing bowl. Drain the thawed frozen spinach really well (I actually squeeze mine) and add it to the Cauli-Rice.

Melt the butter in a medium skillet, over medium-low heat, and sauté the onion until it's just translucent. Add the garlic, sauté for another minute or two, then dump the whole thing in the bowl with the cauliflower and spinach.

Add the eggs, Carb Countdown, salt or Vege-Sal, pepper, and Parmesan and stir the mixture up quite well. Put it in a 1 1/2–2 quart glass (1.5–2 liter) casserole dish that you've sprayed with nonstick cooking spray. Cover the dish with foil and place it in your slow cooker. Pour water around it up to 1" of the rim. Cover the slow cooker, set it to low, and let it cook for 2 1/2 hours.

Open the slow cooker and remove the foil. Sprinkle the mozzarella over your Macadangdang, put the foil back on, recover the pot, and let it cook for another 20 minutes, to melt the cheese. Then turn off the pot, uncover it, take off the foil, and let the whole thing cool just to the point where you can remove it from the water bath without scalding yourself, around 20 more minutes.

**YIELD:** 6 serving each with: 198 calories, 14 g fat, 13 g protein, 5 g carbohydrate, 2 g dietary fiber, 3 g usable carbs.

#  Broccoli with Bacon and Pine Nuts

This is quite special. Don't cook your broccoli any longer than 2 hours!

1 pound (455 grams) frozen broccoli, unthawed

1 clove garlic, crushed

3 slices cooked bacon, crumbled

1 tablespoon (28 grams) butter

1 tablespoon (28 milliliters) oil

2 tablespoons (30 grams) pine nuts (pignolia), toasted

Place the broccoli in your slow cooker. Stir in the garlic and crumble in the bacon. Cover the slow cooker, set it to low, and let it cook for 2 hours.

Before serving, stir in the butter and oil and top with the pine nuts.

**YIELD:** 3 servings, each with: 184 calories, 15 g fat, 8 g protein, 8 g carbohydrate, 5 g dietary fiber, 3 g usable carbs.

# Fauxtatoes

Fauxtatoes is the now nearly-universal name for cauliflower puree, used by low-carbers everywhere as a substitute for mashed potatoes. To make plain Fauxtatoes as a side dish to serve with a slow-cooked main dish, see recipe page 239. These are slow cooked Fauxtatoes with truly tasty additions.

## Cheddar-Barbecue Fauxtatoes

My husband was crazy about these!

1/2 head cauliflower, cut into florets

1/2 cup (120 milliliters) water

1/2 cup (55 grams) shredded cheddar cheese

2 teaspoons Classic Rub (see recipe page 234) or purchased barbecue rub

2 tablespoons (10 grams) Ketatoes mix

Put the cauliflower in your slow cooker, including the stem. Add the water. Cover the slow cooker, set it to high, and let it cook for 3 hours. (Or cook it on low for 5 to 6 hours.)

When the time's up, use a slotted spoon to scoop the cauliflower out of the slow cooker, into your blender or your food processor (have the S-blade in place) and puree it there, or you can drain off the water and use a hand-held blender to puree the cauliflower right in the pot. Either way, drain the cauliflower and puree it!

Stir in everything else, until the cheese has melted.

**YIELD:** 3 servings, each with: 120 calories, 7 g fat, 8 g protein, 6 g carbohydrate, 3 g dietary fiber, 3 g usable carbs.

# Italian Garlic and Herb Fauxtatoes

1/2 head cauliflower, cut into florets

1/2 cup (120 milliliters) chicken broth

1 teaspoon Italian seasoning

1 clove garlic, crushed

1 ounce (28 grams) cream cheese

Guar or xanthan

Place the cauliflower in your slow cooker. Add the broth, Italian seasoning, and garlic. Cover the slow cooker, set it to low, and let it cook for 5 to 6 hours. (Or cook it on high for 3 hours.)

When the time's up, either remove the cauliflower with a slotted spoon and put it in your blender or food processor (with the S-blade in place) and puree it, or drain the broth out of the slow cooker and use a hand-held blender to puree your cauliflower in the pot. Add the cream cheese and stir till melted.

The mixture will still be a little watery. Stir with a whisk as you use guar or xanthan to thicken it up a bit.

**YIELD:** 3 servings, each with: 46 calories, 4 g fat, 2 g protein, 2 g carbohydrate, 1 g dietary fiber, 1 g usable carbs.

# ☺ Ranch and Green Onion Fauxtatoes

This is great with anything with a barbecue flavor.

- 1 head cauliflower, cut into florets
- 1 cup (235 milliliters) water
- 1 cup (100 grams) Ketatoes mix
- 6 teaspoons ranch-style dressing mix
- 4 scallions, thinly sliced

Place the cauliflower in your slow cooker with the water. Cover the slow cooker, set it to low, and let it cook for 5 hours. (Or cook it on high for 3 hours.)

When the time's up, the easiest thing to do is use a hand blender to puree the cauliflower right in the slow cooker. Don't bother to drain the water first. Whisk in the Ketatoes, ranch dressing mix, and scallions.

**YIELD:** 6 servings, each with: 170 calories, 3 g fat, 14 g protein, 23 g carbohydrate, 11 g dietary fiber, 12 g usable carbs.

#  Garlic-Onion Fauxtatoes

Our tester Maria said her kids were particularly impressed by this!

1 head cauliflower, cut into florets

1/2 cup (50 grams) chopped onion

3 cloves garlic, crushed

2/3 cup (150 milliliters) water

2/3 cup (65 grams) Ketatoes mix

3 tablespoons (45 grams) butter

Place the cauliflower in your slow cooker. Add the onion, garlic, and water. Cover the slow cooker, set it to high, and let it cook for 2 1/2 to 3 hours. (Or cook it on low for 5 to 6 hours.)

When the time's up, use a hand-held blender to puree the cauliflower, onion, and garlic right there in the slow cooker. Alternatively, scoop it all into a food processor to puree, but you'll want the water in the pot, so if you transfer the vegetables, put the puree back in the pot with the water when you're done. Now stir in the Ketatoes, butter, and salt and pepper to taste.

**YIELD:** 6 servings, each with: 162 calories, 8 g fat, 9 g protein, 15 g carbohydrate, 7 g dietary fiber, 8 g usable carbs.

# Mashed Turnips

2 large turnips, cubed

1/4 cup (25 grams) chopped onion

3/4 cup (175 milliliters) beef broth

Put the turnips and onion in your slow cooker and add the broth. Cover the slow cooker, set it to low, and let it cook for 6 to 7 hours.

I like to mash these right in the pot with my hand-held blender, but if you prefer you can transfer them to your food processor or regular blender.

If you're going to serve these plain, you might add some butter, salt, and pepper, but if you're serving them with a gravy, they're great as is.

**YIELD:** 4 servings, each with: 31 calories, trace fat, 3 g protein, 5 g carbohydrate, 1 g dietary fiber, 4 g usable carbs.

# Lemon-Parmesan Mushrooms

8 ounces (225 grams) mushrooms

1/2 cup (125 milliliters) chicken broth

1/4 cup (60 milliliters) lemon juice

1/2 cup (40 grams) shredded Parmesan cheese

1/4 cup (16 grams) chopped fresh parsley

Wipe the mushrooms clean with a damp cloth or paper towel, and put 'em in your slow cooker. Pour the broth and lemon juice over them. Cover the slow cooker, set it to low, and let it cook for 6 to 8 hours.

Remove the mushrooms from the slow cooker with a slotted spoon and put them on serving plates. Sprinkle with the Parmesan and parsley.

**YIELD:** 4 servings, each with: 65 calories, 3 g fat, 6 g protein, 5 g carbohydrate, 1 g dietary fiber, 4 g usable carbs.

# Baked Beans

This has a classic baked bean flavor and will be appreciated at any barbecue. I wouldn't attempt this recipe without a slow cooker. Do you have any idea how long it takes to cook soybeans soft? But with your slow cooker, you can just forget about them for 12 hours. If your health food store can't get you black soybeans (they're lower carb than white soybeans) you can order them from www.locarber.com.

2 cups (240 grams) dry black soybeans

2 cups (475 milliliters) water

1/2 cup (50 grams) chopped onion

1/2 tablespoon (7 milliliters) blackstrap molasses

3 tablespoons (25 grams) low-carb ketchup (see recipe page 228)

1 tablespoon dry mustard

2 tablespoons (3 grams) Splenda

2 cups (475 milliliters) water

3/4 pound (340 grams) smoked ham hocks

Put the soybeans in a big, nonreactive bowl and cover with the first 2 cups of water. Let them sit until the water is absorbed. Then put your soaked beans in the freezer overnight. (The freezing water will help break cell walls in the soybeans, making them soften faster when you cook them.)

When you want to cook the soybeans, thaw them, and pour off any soaking water. Put them in your slow cooker. Add the onion, molasses, ketchup, dry mustard, and Splenda. Pour the additional 2 cups of water over all and stir it up. Now dig a hole in the center with a spoon, and plunk the ham hock down in it. Cover the slow cooker, set it to low, and let cook for 12 hours.

Fish out the ham hock with tongs, remove and discard the skin and bone. Chop the meat and stir it back into the beans before serving.

YIELD: 10 servings (5 cups total), each with: 286 calories, 15 g fat, 8 g protein, 12 g carbohydrate, 11 g dietary fiber, 1 g usable carbs.

# Bavarian Cabbage

This is great with the Sauerbrauten on page 89!

- 1 head red cabbage
- 1 medium onion, chopped
- 1 medium Granny Smith apple, chopped
- 6 slices cooked bacon, crumbled
- 2 teaspoons salt
- 1 cup (235 milliliters) water
- 3 tablespoons (4.5 grams) Splenda
- 2/3 cup (150 milliliters) cider vinegar
- 3 tablespoons (45 milliliters) gin

Whack your head of cabbage in quarters, and remove the core. Then whack it into biggish chunks. Put it in a big mixing bowl. Add the onion, apple, and bacon to the cabbage. Toss everything together. Transfer the mixture to your slow cooker. (This will fill a 3-quart jobbie just about to overflowing! I barely got the top on mine.)

In a bowl, mix together the salt, water, Splenda, vinegar, and gin. Pour the mixture over the cabbage. Cover the slow cooker, set it to low, and let it cook for 6 to 8 hours.

**YIELD:** 6 servings, each with: 80 calories, 3 g fat, 2 g protein, 7 g carbohydrate, 1 g dietary fiber, 6 g usable carbs.

# Slow Cooker Chutney

This is the slow cooker version of my Major Gray's Chutney recipe from *500 More Low-Carb Recipes*. It's wonderful with anything curried.

2 pounds (1 kilogram) sliced peaches

1/3 cup (30 grams) ginger root slices

1 1/2 cups (35 grams) Splenda

3 cloves garlic

1 teaspoon red pepper flakes

1 teaspoon cloves

1 1/2 cups (355 milliliters) cider vinegar

Guar or xanthan

Combine everything but the guar or xanthan in your slow cooker. Cover the slow cooker, set it to low, and let it cook for 4 hours.

Take the lid off and let it cook for another hour, to let it cook down. Thicken a bit more, if you like, and store in an airtight container in the fridge.

**YIELD:** 32 servings (1 quart total), each with: 15 calories, trace fat, trace protein, 4 g carbohydrate, 1 g dietary fiber, 3 g usable carbs.

# Slow Cooker Cranberry Sauce

I like to have cranberry sauce on hand for those occasions when I don't want to do much cooking. It adds interest to plain roasted chicken (or even store-bought rotisseried chicken.) It's easy to do, and makes plenty!

- 24 ounces (670 grams) cranberries
- 1 cup (235 milliliters) water
- 2 cups (50 grams) Splenda

Simply combine everything in your slow cooker and give it a stir. Cover the slow cooker, set it to low, and let it cook for 3 hours.

This won't be as syrupy as commercial cranberry sauce because of the lack of sugar. If this bothers you, you can thicken your sauce with your trusty guar or xanthan shaker, but I generally leave mine as is. This makes quite a lot, so divide it between three or four snap-top containers, and store it in the freezer. This way, you'll have cranberry sauce on hand whenever you bring home a rotisseried chicken!

**YIELD:** Makes about 2 3/4 cups, or 22 servings of 2 tablespoons, each with: 15 calories, trace fat, trace protein, 4 g carbohydrate, 1 g dietary fiber, 3 g usable carbs.

# Cranberry-Peach Chutney

This is seriously kicked-up from regular cranberry sauce! It's a natural with curried poultry, but try it with any simple poultry or pork dish.

12 ounces (340 grams) cranberries

1 1/2 cups (330 grams) diced peaches

    (I use unsweetened frozen peach slices, diced.)

1 clove garlic, minced

3 inches (76 millimeters) ginger root, sliced into paper-thin rounds

1 lime, sliced paper-thin

1 1/4 cups (30 grams) Splenda

1 cinnamon stick

1 teaspoon mustard seed

1/4 teaspoon salt

1/4 teaspoon orange extract

1/4 teaspoon baking soda

Combine everything but the baking soda in your slow cooker. Cover the slow cooker, set it to low, and let it cook for 3 hours, stirring once halfway through.

When the time's up, stir in the baking soda and keep stirring till the fizzing subsides. Store in a tightly lidded container in the fridge. If you plan to keep it for long, freezing's a good idea.

Why baking soda? Because by neutralizing some of the acid in the cranberries, it lets you get away with less Splenda—and fewer carbs.

**YIELD:** Makes about 2 1/2 cups, or 20 servings of 2 tablespoons, each with: 31 calories, trace fat, trace protein, 8 g carbohydrate, 1 g dietary fiber, 7 g usable carbs.

# CHAPTER ELEVEN

# Slow Cooker Desserts

There are desserts that adapt well to the slow cooker, and then there are desserts that don't. In this chapter, I've really played to the slow cooker's strengths. Custards actually cook better in a slow cooker than in the oven, which is why you'll find half a dozen of them here. Indeed, they're so easy in the slow cooker, and so appealing and nutritious, you may find yourself making custard more often.

Your slow cooker also excels at baking cheesecake, though you may not know it yet. Give it a try!

# ⛖ Chocolate Fudge Custard

This really is dense and fudgy. It's intensely chocolatey, too.

> 1 cup (235 milliliters) Carb Countdown dairy beverage
>
> 3 ounces (85 grams) unsweetened baking chocolate
>
> 2/3 cup (16 grams) Splenda
>
> 1 cup (235 milliliters) heavy cream
>
> 1/2 teaspoon vanilla extract
>
> 1 pinch salt
>
> 6 eggs, beaten

In a saucepan, over the lowest possible heat (use a double boiler or heat diffuser if you have one) warm the Carb Countdown with the chocolate. When the chocolate melts, whisk the two together, then whisk in the Splenda.

Spray a 6-cup glass casserole dish with nonstick cooking spray. Pour the cream into it and add the chocolate mixture. Whisk in the vanilla extract and salt. Now add the eggs, one by one, whisking each in well before adding the next one.

Put the casserole dish in your slow cooker and pour water around it, up to 1" of the top rim. Cover the slow cooker, set it to low, and let it cook for 4 hours.

Then turn off the slow cooker, remove the lid, and let the water cool enough so it won't scald you before removing the casserole dish. Chill the custard well before serving.

YIELD: 6 servings, each with: 299 calories, 28 g fat, 10 g protein, 6 g carbohydrate, 2 g dietary fiber, 4 g usable carbs.

# Flan

This is my slow cooker version of Maria's Flan from *500 Low-Carb Recipes*. Rich!

2 tablespoons (40 grams) sugar-free imitation honey

1 teaspoon blackstrap molasses

1 cup (235 milliliters) Carb Countdown dairy beverage

1 cup (235 milliliters) heavy cream

6 eggs

2/3 cup (16 grams) Splenda

1 teaspoon vanilla

1 pinch nutmeg

1 pinch salt

Spray a 6-cup glass casserole dish with nonstick cooking spray. In a bowl, mix together the honey and the molasses. Pour the mixture in the bottom of the casserole dish.

In a mixing bowl, preferably one with a pouring lip, combine the Carb Countdown, cream, eggs, Splenda, vanilla, nutmeg, and salt. Whisk everything together well. Pour the mixture into the casserole dish.

Carefully lower the casserole dish into your slow cooker. Now pour water around the casserole dish, to within 1" of the rim. Cover the slow cooker, set it to low, and let it cook for 3 to 3 1/2 hours.

**YIELD:** 6 servings, each with: 229 calories, 20 g fat, 8 g protein, 3 g carbohydrate, trace dietary fiber, 3 g usable carbs.

# Southeast Asian Coconut Custard

I adapted this from a carby recipe in another slow cooker book. Maria, who tested it, says it's wonderful and also has a Latino feel to it. Look for shredded unsweetened coconut in Asian markets and health food stores.

1/4 cup (5 grams) sugar-free imitation honey

1/2 teaspoon blackstrap molasses

1 1/2 teaspoons grated ginger root

1 tablespoon (14 milliliters) lime juice

14 ounces (425 milliliters) coconut milk

2/3 cup (16 grams) Splenda

1/4 teaspoon ground cardamom

1 teaspoon grated ginger root

1/2 cup (120 milliliters) Carb Countdown dairy beverage

1/2 cup (120 milliliters) heavy cream

1/2 teaspoon vanilla extract

4 eggs

1/2 cup (35 grams) shredded unsweetened coconut

Spray a 6-cup glass casserole dish with nonstick cooking spray. Put the honey and molasses in the casserole dish. Cover the casserole dish with plastic wrap or a plate and microwave on high for 2 minutes. Add the 1 1/2 teaspoons ginger and lime juice and stir. Set aside.

In a mixing bowl, combine the coconut milk, Splenda, cardamom, 1 teaspoon ginger, Carb Countdown, cream, vanilla extract, and eggs. Whisk until well combined. Pour into the casserole dish. Cover the casserole dish with foil and secure it with a rubber band.

Put the casserole dish in your slow cooker and pour water around it, to within 1" of the rim. Cover the slow cooker, set it to low, and let it cook for 3 to 4 hours.

Turn off the slow cooker, uncover, and let it cool till you can lift out the casserole dish without scalding your fingers. Chill overnight.

Before serving, stir the coconut in a dry skillet over medium heat until it's golden. Remove the custard from the fridge and run a knife carefully around the edge. Put a plate on top and carefully invert the custard onto the plate. Sprinkle the toasted coconut on top.

**YIELD:** 8 servings, each with: 227 calories, 22 g fat, 5 g protein, 5 g carbohydrate, 2 g dietary fiber, 3 g usable carbs.

# Maple Custard

This is for all you maple fans out there, and I know you are legion!

1 1/2 cups (355 milliliters) Carb Countdown dairy beverage

1/2 cup (120 milliliters) heavy cream

1/3 cup (78 milliliters) sugar-free pancake syrup

1/3 cup (8 grams) Splenda

3 eggs

1 pinch salt

1 teaspoon vanilla extract

1/2 teaspoon maple extract

Simply whisk everything together and pour the mixture into a 6-cup glass casserole dish you've sprayed with nonstick cooking spray. Put the casserole dish in your slow cooker and pour water around it to within 1" of the rim. Cover the slow cooker, set it to low, and let it cook for 4 hours.

When the time's up, turn off the slow cooker, remove the lid, and let it sit until the water is cool enough so that you can remove the casserole without risk of scalding. Chill well before serving.

**YIELD:** 6 servings, each with: 135 calories, 12 g fat, 6 g protein, 2 g carbohydrate, 0 g dietary fiber, 2 g usable carbs. (Counts do not include polyols in pancake syrup.)

# Maple-Pumpkin Custard

This is very much like the filling of a pumpkin pie, without the crust. The pecans add a little textural contrast.

15 ounces (430 grams) canned pumpkin

1 cup (235 milliliters) Carb Countdown dairy beverage

1/2 cup (120 milliliters) heavy cream

1/3 cup (78 milliliters) sugar-free pancake syrup

1/3 cup (8 grams) Splenda

1/2 teaspoon maple flavoring

3 eggs

1 pinch salt

1 tablespoon (6 grams) pumpkin pie spice

1/3 cup (35 grams) chopped pecans

1 1/2 teaspoons butter

Whipped Topping (see recipe page 238)

In a mixing bowl, preferably one with a pouring lip, whisk together the pumpkin, Carb Countdown, cream, pancake syrup, Splenda, maple flavoring, eggs, salt, and pumpkin pie spice.

Spray a 6-cup glass casserole dish with nonstick cooking spray. Pour the custard mixture into it. Place it in your slow cooker. Now carefully fill the space around the casserole with water, up to 1" from the rim. Cover the slow cooker, set it to low, and let it cook for 3 to 4 hours.

Remove the lid, turn off the slow cooker, and let it cool till you can remove the casserole dish without scalding your fingers. Chill the custard for at least several hours.

Before serving, put the pecans and butter in a heavy skillet over medium heat and stir them for 5 minutes or so. Set aside. Also have the Whipped Topping made and standing by.

Serve the custard with a dollop of Whipped Topping and 1 tablespoon of toasted pecans on each serving.

**YIELD:** 6 servings, each with: 341 calories, 31 g fat, 7 g protein, 10 g carbohydrate, 3 g dietary fiber, 7 g usable carbs.

# Apricot Custard

Don't go increasing the quantity of apricot preserves here. They're the biggest source of carbs. This dessert is yummy, though!

1/3 cup (105 grams) low-sugar apricot preserves

2 tablespoons (28 milliliters) lemon juice

2 teaspoons Splenda

1 1/2 cups (355 milliliters) Carb Countdown dairy beverage

1/2 cup (120 milliliters) heavy cream

4 eggs

2/3 cup (16 grams) Splenda

1/2 teaspoon almond extract

1 pinch salt

Whisk together the preserves, lemon juice, and the 2 teaspoons of Splenda. Spread them over the bottom of a 6-cup glass casserole dish you've sprayed with nonstick cooking spray. Set aside.

Whisk together the Carb Countdown, cream, eggs, 2/3 cup Splenda, almond extract, and salt. Pour into the prepared casserole gently, so as not to mix in the apricot preserves.

Place the casserole dish in your slow cooker. Pour water around the casserole to within 1" of the rim. Cover the slow cooker, set it to low, and let it cook for 4 hours.

When the time's up, turn off the slow cooker, uncover it, and let it cool until you can remove the casserole dish without risk of scalding. Chill well before serving.

**YIELD:** 6 servings, each with: 165 calories, 12 g fat, 7 g protein, 7 g carbohydrate, trace dietary fiber, 7 g usable carbs.

# Peaches with Butterscotch Sauce

These are delectable. You can serve them as is, with a little heavy cream, with Whipped Topping (see recipe page 238) — or, the Big Casino, with a scoop of low-carb vanilla ice cream.

1 pound (455 grams) frozen, unsweetened, sliced peaches

2 teaspoons lemon juice

1/3 cup (8 grams) Splenda

2 tablespoons (40 grams) sugar-free imitation honey

1/2 teaspoon blackstrap molasses

2 tablespoons (28 milliliters) heavy cream

1/4 teaspoon cinnamon

2 tablespoons (28 grams) butter, melted

Guar or xanthan

Place the peaches in your slow cooker. (I didn't even bother to thaw mine.)

In a bowl, stir together the lemon juice, Splenda, honey, molasses, cream, cinnamon, and butter. Pour the mixture over the peaches. Cover the slow cooker, set it to low, and let it cook for 6 hours.

Thicken the sauce to a creamy consistency with a little guar or xanthan and serve hot.

YIELD: 6 servings, each with: 86 calories, 6 g fat, 1 g protein, 9 g carbohydrate, 2 g dietary fiber, 7 g usable carbs. (Analysis does not include polyols.)

# ⬚ Rhubarb Flummery

Because it's so sour, rhubarb is low-carb. This is a simple, old-fashioned dessert.

> 1 pound (455 grams) frozen rhubarb
> 1/2 cup (12 grams) Splenda
> 1/2 cup (120 milliliters) water
> 1/8 teaspoon orange extract
> Guar or xanthan

Place the rhubarb in your slow cooker and stir in the Splenda, water, and orange extract. Cover the slow cooker, set it to low, and let it cook for 5 to 6 hours.

When the time's up, the rhubarb will be very soft. Mash it with a fork to a rough pulp. Thicken the sauce to a soft pudding consistency with guar or xanthan and serve hot or cold.

This dessert is great with a little heavy cream or Whipped Topping (see recipe page 238).

YIELD: 6 servings, each with: 16 calories, trace fat, trace protein, 4 g carbohydrate, 1 g dietary fiber, 3 g usable carbs.

# Hot Cinnamon Mocha

Assemble this in your slow cooker before going skating, caroling, or to a football game, and have a winter party waiting when you get home!

1/2 gallon (1.75 liters) chocolate-flavored Carb Countdown dairy beverage

2 cinnamon sticks

3 tablespoons (8 grams) instant coffee granules

1 1/2 teaspoons vanilla extract

Combine everything in your slow cooker and give it a stir. Cover the slow cooker, set it to high, and let it cook for 3 hours. Turn the slow cooker to low and serve from the slow cooker.

If it's a grown-up party, put a bottle of Mockahlua on the side for spiking! (See recipe page 238.)

**YIELD:** 10 servings, each with: 92 calories, 4 g fat, 10 g protein, 5 g carbohydrate, 2 g dietary fiber, 3 g usable carbs.

# About Cheesecake

There were so many cheesecake recipes in *500 More Low-Carb Recipes* that I only did three for this book. However, cheesecake works very well in the slow cooker, so feel free to experiment with baking your favorite low-carb cheesecake recipes this way.

You'll notice I've called for light cream cheese (or Neufchâtel, which is, so far as I can tell, the same thing) and light sour cream in these recipes, instead of the full-fat versions. There's a reason for this: The light versions generally have no more carbohydrate than their full-fat counterparts, and they are, of course, lower calorie. I consider that a gain, and the cheesecakes come out very well. However, feel free to use the full-fat versions if you prefer.

# Mochaccino Cheesecake

This cheesecake is extraordinary, as good as any dessert I ever had in a restaurant. This alone is a good enough reason to go buy a large, round slow cooker, and an 8" springform to fit into it! It's also a good excuse to make some Mockahlua, but who needs an excuse to do that?

Crisp Chocolate Crust (see recipe on the next page)
16 ounces (455 grams) light cream cheese or Neufchâtel cheese, softened
1 egg
1/4 cup (60 milliliters) heavy cream
1/2 cup (40 grams) + 2 tablespoons (11 grams) unsweetened cocoa powder
1/2 cup (12 grams) Splenda
1/4 cup (60 milliliters) Mockahlua (see recipe page 238)
2 tablespoons (28 milliliters) brewed coffee

Using your electric mixer, beat together the cream cheese, egg, and cream until quite smooth. (You'll need to scrape down the sides of the bowl several times.) Now beat in the cocoa powder, Splenda, Mockahlua, and coffee. When it's all well blended and very smooth, pour into the crust. Cover the springform pan tightly with foil, squeezing it in around the rim.

Take a big sheet of foil, at least 18" (46 centimeters) long, and roll it into a loose cylinder. Bend it into a circle and place it in the bottom of your slow cooker. (You're making a rack to put the pan on.) Pour 1/4" of water in the bottom of the slow cooker, then put the pan on the donut of foil. Cover the slow cooker, set it to high, and let it cook for 3 to 4 hours.

Turn off the slow cooker, uncover, and let cool for at least 20 to 30 minutes before you try to remove the pan from the slow cooker. Chill well before serving.

It's nice to make the Whipped Topping (see recipe page 238), with a little Mockahlua in it, to serve on top of this, but it's hardly essential.

**YIELD:** 12 servings, each with: 284 calories, 24 g fat, 11 g protein, 10 g carbohydrate, 4 g dietary fiber, 6 g usable carbs. (Analysis includes Crisp Chocolate Crust. You could cut this into eight, more generous servings if you'd like.)

# Crisp Chocolate Crust

1 1/2 cups (220 grams) almonds

1/4 cup (6 grams) Splenda

2 squares bitter chocolate, melted

3 tablespoons (45 grams) butter, melted

2 tablespoons (16 grams) vanilla whey protein powder

Preheat the oven to 325°F.

Using the S-blade of your food processor, grind the almonds until they're the texture of corn meal. Add the Splenda and pulse to combine. Pour in the chocolate and butter and run processor till evenly distributed. (You may need to stop the processor and run the tip of a knife blade around the outer edge to get everything to combine properly.) Then add the protein powder and pulse again to combine.

Turn the mixture into an 8" springform pan you've coated with nonstick cooking spray. Press firmly and evenly into place. Bake for 10 to 12 minutes in the preheated oven. Cool before filling.

**YIELD:** 12 servings, each with: 164 calories, 15 g fat, 6 g protein, 5 g carbohydrate, 3 g dietary fiber, 2 g usable carbs.

# New York–Style Cheesecake

You can top this with fruit if you like, but it's mighty good just as it is.

"Graham" Crust (see recipe on the next page)
1 pound (455 grams) light cream cheese or Neufchâtel cheese, softened
1/2 cup (120 grams) light sour cream
2 eggs
1/2 cup (12 grams) Splenda
2 teaspoons vanilla extract
1 pinch salt

Prepare the "Graham" Crust and let it cool.

Using your electric mixer, beat the cheese, sour cream, and eggs until they're very smooth. (You'll need to scrape down the sides of the bowl at least a few times.) Now beat in the Splenda, vanilla extract, and salt. Pour into the waiting crust. Cover the pan tightly with foil, squeezing it in around the rim.

Take a big sheet of foil, at least 18" (45 centimeters) long, and roll it into a loose cylinder. Bend it into a circle, and place it in the bottom of your slow cooker. (You're making a rack to put the pan on.) Pour 1/4" of water into your slow cooker, then put the pan on the donut of foil. Cover the slow cooker, set it to high, and let it cook for 3 to 4 hours.

Turn off the slow cooker, uncover, and let cool for at least 20 to 30 minutes before you try to remove the pan from the slow cooker. Chill well before serving.

**YIELD:** 12 servings, each with: 241 calories, 21 g fat, 8 g protein, 6 g carbohydrate, 2 g dietary fiber, 4 g usable carbs. (You could cut this into eight, more generous servings if you'd like.)

#  "Graham" Crust

Wheat germ and wheat bran give this a "graham" flavor.

  1 1/4 cups (180 grams) almonds

  2 tablespoons (14 grams) wheat germ

  2 tablespoons (14 grams) wheat bran

  3 tablespoons (4.5 grams) Splenda

  1 pinch salt

  6 tablespoons (80 grams) butter, melted

Preheat the oven to 325°F.

Put the almonds in your food processor with the S-blade in place. Run it until they're ground to about the texture of corn meal. Add the wheat germ, wheat bran, Splenda, and salt and pulse to combine. Now turn on the processor and pour in the butter, running the processor until everything's well combined. (You may need to stop the processor and run a knife around the bottom edge to make sure all the dry ingredients come in contact with the butter.)

Turn this mixture out into an 8" springform pan you've sprayed with nonstick cooking spray. Press firmly into place. Bake for 10 to 12 minutes, or until just turning gold around the edges. Cool before filling.

**YIELD:** 12 servings, each with: 144 calories, 14 g fat, 3 g protein, 4 g carbohydrate, 2 g dietary fiber, 2 g usable carbs.

# Peanut Butter Cheesecake

You can certainly eat this plain, but I'd likely top it with some sugar-free chocolate sauce. Sorbee makes one that's available in my grocery store, or you could order some from a low-carb e-tailer. Or you could make some from the recipe on page 237. Or, for that matter, you could melt 6 to 8 ounces (170 to 225 grams) of your favorite sugar-free chocolate bars and swirl them into the peanut butter batter before baking. The possibilities are endless!

Crisp Chocolate Crust (see recipe page 222) or "Graham" Crust >>>>..
  (see recipe page 224)
16 ounces (455 grams) light cream cheese or Neufchâtel cheese, softened
1/2 cup (120 grams) light sour cream
1 egg
3/4 cup (200 grams) natural peanut butter
  (salted is better than no-salt-added, here)
2/3 cup (16 grams) Splenda
1/2 teaspoons blackstrap molasses

Have your crust made and standing by.

Using your electric mixer, beat the cream cheese or Neufchâtel, sour cream, and egg until they're very smooth. (You'll want to scrape down the sides of the bowl several times.) Now beat in the peanut butter, Splenda, and molasses.

When the mixture is very smooth and well blended, pour it into the crust. Cover the pan tightly with foil, squeezing it in around the rim.

Take a big sheet of foil, at least 18" (45 centimeters) long, and roll it into a loose cylinder. Bend it into a circle, and place it in the bottom of your slow cooker. (You're making a rack to put the pan on.) Pour 1/4" of water into the slow cooker, then put the pan on the donut of foil. Cover the slow cooker, set it to high, and let it cook for 3 to 4 hours.

Turn off the slow cooker, uncover, and let cool for at least 20 to 30 minutes before you try to remove the pan from the slow cooker. Chill well before serving.

**YIELD:** 12 servings, each with: 364 calories, 32 g fat, 13 g protein, 10 g carbohydrate, 4 g dietary fiber, 6 g usable carbs. (Analysis includes Crisp Chocolate Crust. Analysis does not include any chocolate sauce or melted chocolate you might add! You could cut this into eight, more generous servings if you'd like.)

# CHAPTER TWELVE

# Just A Few Extras...

This is where I've tucked the recipes that you need to make other recipes, but that aren't, themselves, slow cooker stuff. It just seemed easiest to put them all in one place, you know? Most of these have appeared in one or more of my previous cookbooks. And by the way, we didn't count these toward your grand total of 200 slow cooker recipes—that's why they're extras.

# Dana's No-Sugar Ketchup

This recipe has appeared in all my cookbooks because ketchup is an essential ingredient in so many recipes, but store-bought ketchup usually has so much sugar. Recently, commercially-made low-carb ketchup has been appearing in the grocery stores. If you can get this, do so because food processors can get ingredients the home cook cannot, so store-bought low-carb ketchup is lower in carbs than this. If you can't find low-carb ketchup, however, this is easy to make, tastes great, and is about half the carbs of regular ketchup. Be aware that recipes that list ketchup as an ingredient are analyzed for this homemade version, so if you use commercial low-carb ketchup, the carb counts will be a tad lower.

6 ounces (95 grams) tomato paste

2/3 cup (150 milliliters) cider vinegar

1/3 cup (75 milliliters) water

1/3 cup (8 grams) Splenda

2 tablespoons (20 grams) minced onion

2 cloves garlic

1 teaspoon salt

1/8 teaspoon ground allspice

1/8 teaspoon ground cloves

1/8 teaspoon pepper

Put everything in your blender and run it until the onion disappears. Scrape it into a container with a tight lid and store it in the refrigerator.

**YIELD:** Makes roughly 1 1/2 cups, or 12 servings of 2 tablespoons, each with: 15 calories, trace fat, 1 g protein, 5 g carbohydrate, 1 g fiber, 4 g usable carbs.

#  Cocktail Sauce

You'll need this for the Easy Party Shrimp on page 24!

> $1/2$ cup (120 grams) Dana's No-Sugar Ketchup (page 228)
>   or purchased low-carb ketchup
> 2 teaspoons prepared horseradish
> $1/4$ teaspoon Tabasco sauce
> 1 teaspoon lemon juice

Combine all ingredients in a bowl and mix well.

**YIELD:** Makes about $1/2$ cup. The whole batch contains: 142 calories, 1 g fat, 5 g protein, 36 g carbohydrate, 6 g dietary fiber, 30 g usable carbs. Good thing you'll be sharing it! You can drop this carb count considerably by using commercially-made low-carb ketchup.

# Florida Sunshine Tangerine Barbecue Sauce

The name of this sauce is partly from the tangerine note, which is unusual and delicious, but the name is also from the fact that this sauce is at least as hot as the Florida sun! It's especially good on poultry. You can use this in any of the recipes that call for barbecue sauce, or you can use the Kansas City–style sauce on the following page—this one's lower carb, but less traditional. Or, for that matter, you can use the newly available bottled low-carb barbecue sauce. You won't hurt my feelings.

12 ounces (355 milliliters) Diet Rite Tangerine Soda

1/4 cup (6 grams) Splenda

1 tablespoon (7 grams) chili powder

2 teaspoons black pepper

1 teaspoon ginger

1 teaspoon dry mustard

1 teaspoon onion salt

4 cloves garlic, crushed

1/2 teaspoon cayenne

1/2 teaspoon coriander

1/2 teaspoon red pepper flakes

1 bay leaf

1/2 cup (120 milliliters) cider vinegar

1 tablespoon (20 grams) sugar-free imitation honey

1 tablespoon (14 milliliters) Worcestershire sauce

3/4 cup (180 grams) Dana's No-Sugar Ketchup (page 228) or purchased low-carb ketchup

Pour the soda into a nonreactive saucepan and turn the heat under it to medium-low. While that's heating, measure the other ingredients into the sauce. By the time you get to the ketchup, it should be simmering. Whisk everything together until smooth and let it simmer over lowest heat for a good 10 to 15 minutes.

**YIELD:** Makes about 3 cups, or 24 servings of 2 tablespoons, each with: 11 calories, trace fat, trace protein, 3 g carbohydrate, trace dietary fiber, 3 g usable carbs.

# ☐ Dana's "Kansas City" Barbecue Sauce

This recipe, from *The Low-Carb Barbecue Book*, is it—what most of us think of when we think of barbecue sauce: tomato-y, spicy, and sweet. It's unbelievably close to a top-flight commercial barbecue sauce—and my Kansas City–raised husband agrees. If you like a smoky note in your barbecue sauce, add 1 teaspoon of liquid smoke flavoring to this. (Note: If you can get it locally, commercially-made low-carb barbecue sauce is likely to be lower carb than this recipe.)

   2 tablespoons (28 grams) butter

   1 clove garlic

   1/4 cup (25 grams) chopped onion

   1 tablespoon (14 milliliters) lemon juice

   1 cup (240 grams) Dana's No-Sugar Ketchup (page 228) or purchased
      low-carb ketchup

   1/3 cup (8 grams) Splenda

   1 tablespoon (20 grams) blackstrap molasses

   2 tablespoons (28 milliliters) Worcestershire sauce

   1 tablespoon (9 grams) chili powder

   1 tablespoon (14 milliliters) white vinegar

   1 teaspoon pepper

   1/4 teaspoon salt

Combine everything in a saucepan over low heat. Heat until the butter melts, stir the whole thing up, and let it simmer for 5 minutes or so. That's it!

**YIELD:** Roughly 1 3/4 cups, or 14 servings of 2 tablespoons each, each with: 45 calories, 3 g fat, 1 g protein, 7 g carbohydrate, 1 g fiber, 6 g usable carbs.

# Piedmont Mustard Sauce

This bright-yellow sauce, heavy on the mustard, but completely free of tomato, is typical of the Piedmont region of North Carolina. Try it on Slow Cooker Pulled Pork (see recipe page 142).

1/2 cup (125 grams) yellow mustard

2 tablespoons (28 milliliters) lemon juice

2 tablespoons (3 grams) Splenda

1 tablespoon (14 milliliters) white vinegar

1/4 teaspoon cayenne

Combine everything in a saucepan and simmer for 5 minutes over low heat.

**YIELD:** Makes roughly 3/4 cup, or 6 servings of 2 tablespoons, each with: 17 calories, 1 g fat, 1 g protein, 2 g carbohydrate, 1 g dietary fiber, 1 g usable carbs.

# Eastern Carolina Vinegar Sauce

This is the traditional Eastern Carolina sauce for pulled pork. It's just sweetened vinegar with a good hint of hot pepper. It'll be great with your Slow Cooker Pulled Pork (see recipe page 142)!

1/2 cup (120 milliliters) cider vinegar

1 1/2 tablespoons (2 grams) Splenda

1/4 teaspoon blackstrap molasses

1 teaspoon red pepper flakes

1/4 teaspoon cayenne

Combine everything in a saucepan and simmer for 5 minutes over low heat.

**YIELD:** 6 servings, each with: 4 calories, trace fat, trace protein, 2 g carbohydrate, trace dietary fiber, 2 g usable carbs.

# Hoisin Sauce

Hoisin sauce is sort of Chinese barbecue sauce, and it customarily contains a lot of sugar. It also doesn't usually have peanut butter in it, but it works quite well here. This is a repeat from *500 Low-Carb Recipes*, by the way.

4 tablespoons (60 milliliters) soy sauce

2 tablespoons (32 grams) natural peanut butter

2 tablespoons (3 grams) Splenda

2 teaspoons white vinegar

1 clove garlic

2 teaspoons dark sesame oil

1/8 teaspoon five-spice powder

Just assemble everything in your blender and blend till it's smooth. Store it in a tightly lidded jar in the fridge. Feel free to double or triple this, if you like.

**YIELD:** Makes roughly 1/3 cup, or 6 servings of about 1 tablespoon, each with: 52 calories, 4 g fat , 2 g protein, 2 g carbohydrate, trace dietary fiber, 1 g usable carbs.

# Low-Carb Teriyaki Sauce

There's now commercial low-carb teriyaki sauce on the market, but I like this better, and it's so easy to make, why wouldn't I? Why wouldn't you?

1/2 cup (120 milliliters) soy sauce

1/4 cup (60 milliliters) dry sherry

1 clove garlic, crushed

2 tablespoons (3 grams) Splenda

1 tablespoon (8 grams) grated ginger root

Combine all the ingredients. Refrigerate until ready to use.

**YIELD:** Makes 3/4 cup, or 12 servings of 1 tablespoon, each with: 13 calories, trace fat, 1 g protein, 1 g carbohydrate, trace dietary fiber, 1 g usable carbs.

# Classic Rub

This barbecue rub first appeared in *The Low-Carb Barbecue Book*, and it's a great choice in any recipe that calls for barbecue rub.

1/4 cup (6 grams) Splenda

1 tablespoon (18 grams) seasoned salt

1 tablespoon (8 grams) garlic powder

1 tablespoon (18 grams) celery salt

1 tablespoon (9 grams) onion powder

2 tablespoons (14 grams) paprika

1 tablespoon (9 grams) chili powder

2 teaspoons pepper

1 teaspoon lemon pepper

1 teaspoon ground sage

1 teaspoon mustard

1/2 teaspoon thyme

1/2 teaspoon cayenne

Simply stir everything together and store in an airtight container.

**YIELD:** Makes 13 tablespoons of rub, each with: 13 calories, trace fat, 1 g protein, 2 g carbohydrate, 1 g dietary fiber, 1 g usable carbs.

#  Cajun Seasoning

This New Orleans–style seasoning, originally from *500 Low-Carb Recipes*, is good sprinkled over chicken, steak, pork, fish—just about anything. It will also work in any recipe in this book that calls for Cajun seasoning. But if you'd rather use purchased seasoning, go for it.

2 1/2 tablespoons (18 grams) paprika

2 tablespoons (30 grams) salt

2 tablespoons (16 grams) garlic powder

1 tablespoon (6 grams) pepper

1 tablespoon (9 grams) onion powder

1 tablespoon (5 grams) cayenne

1 tablespoon (4 grams) dried oregano

1 tablespoon (3 grams) dried thyme

Combine all ingredients thoroughly and store in an airtight container.

**YIELD:** Makes 2/3 cup. The whole batch contains: 187 calories, 4 g fat, 8 g protein, 37 g carbohydrate, 9 g dietary fiber, 28 g usable carbs. (Considering how spicy this is, you're unlikely to use more than a teaspoon or two at a time. One teaspoon has 1 gram of carbohydrate, with a trace of fiber.)

# Adobo Seasoning

Adobo is a popular seasoning in Latin America and the Caribbean. It's available at many grocery stores, in the spice aisle or the international aisle. But if you can't find it, it sure is easy to make.

10 teaspoons garlic powder

5 teaspoons dried oregano

5 teaspoons pepper

2 1/2 teaspoons paprika

5 teaspoons salt

Simply measure everything into a bowl, stir, and store in a lidded shaker jar.

**YIELD:** Makes a little over 1/2 cup, or about 48 servings of 1/2 teaspoon, each with: 3 calories, trace fat, trace protein, 1g carbohydrate, trace dietary fiber, 1 g usable carbs.

# Garam Masala

This is an Indian spice blend used in several of the curries in this book. You may well be able to buy perfectly lovely garam masala already made at a local Asian market or big grocery store—I can! But if you can't, you can easily make your own.

2 tablespoons (6 grams) ground cumin

2 tablespoons (10 grams) ground coriander

2 tablespoons (6 grams) ground cardamom

1 1/2 tablespoons black pepper

4 teaspoons ground cinnamon

1/2 teaspoon ground cloves

1 teaspoon ground nutmeg

Simply combine everything and store in an airtight container.

**YIELD:** Makes roughly 9 tablespoons, each with: 19 calories, 1 g fat, 1 g protein, 4 g carbohydrate, 1 g dietary fiber, 3 g usable carbs.

# Sugar-Free Chocolate Sauce

This is as good as any sugar-based chocolate sauce you've ever had, if I do say so myself. Which I do. Don't try to make this with Splenda; it won't work. The polyol sweetener somehow makes the water and the chocolate combine. It's chemistry, or magic, or some darned thing. You very likely will need to order maltitol. Just Web search under "low carbohydrate," and you'll find dozens of Web sites ready to ship anything your heart desires. My favorite is Carb Smart.

1/3 cup (75 milliliters) water

2 ounces (4 tablespoons) unsweetened baking chocolate

1/2 cup (100 grams) maltitol

3 tablespoons (45 grams) butter

1/4 teaspoon vanilla

Put the water and chocolate in a glass measuring cup and microwave on high for 1 to 1 1/2 minutes, or until the chocolate has melted. Stir in the maltitol and microwave on high for another 3 minutes, stirring halfway through. Stir in the butter and vanilla.

**NOTE:** This works beautifully with maltitol. However, when I tried to make it with other granular polyols—erythritol, isomalt—it started out fine but crystallized and turned grainy as it cooled. I'd stick with maltitol.

**YIELD:** Makes roughly 1 cup, or 8 servings of 2 tablespoons, each with: 75 calories, 8 g fat, 1 g protein, 2 g carbohydrate, 1 g dietary fiber, 1 g usable carbs. (This does not include the maltitol.)

# ⬚ Mockahlua

This recipe originally appeared in *500 Low-Carb Recipes*, but because I've included it in some recipes in the dessert chapter I thought I'd better repeat it! This recipe makes quite a lot, but don't worry about that; 100-proof vodka's a darned good preservative. Your Mockahlua will keep indefinitely.

2 1/2 cups (355 milliliters) water

3 cups (75 grams) Splenda

3 tablespoons (8 grams) instant coffee granules

1 teaspoon vanilla extract

1 bottle (750 milliliters) 100-proof vodka (Use the cheap stuff.)

In a large pitcher or measuring cup, combine the water, Splenda, coffee granules, and vanilla extract. Stir until the coffee and Splenda are completely dissolved.

Pour the mixture through a funnel into a 1.5 or 2 liter bottle. (A clean 1.5 liter wine bottle works fine, so long as you've saved the cork.) Pour in the vodka. Cork and shake well.

**YIELD:** 32 servings of 1 1/2 ounces—a standard "shot," each with: 53 calories, 0 g fat, trace protein, trace carbohydrate, 0 g dietary fiber, trace usable carbs.


# ⬚ Whipped Topping

I keep repeating this recipe, but then, it's a wonderful, classic whipped cream topping for any dessert.

1 cup (235 milliliters) heavy cream, chilled

3 teaspoons sugar-free vanilla instant pudding mix

Simply whip the cream with the pudding mix. Use your electric mixer, or, if you like, a whisk—neither a blender nor a food processor will work. Stop whipping as soon as your topping is nice and thick, or you'll end up with vanilla butter!

If you make this ahead of time, refrigerate it until you're ready to serve dessert.

**YIELD:** 8 servings, each with: 104 calories, 11 g fat, 1 g protein, 1 g carbohydrate, 0 g dietary fiber, 1 g usable carbs.

## Cauli-Rice

With thanks to Fran McCullough! I got this idea from her book *Living Low-Carb*, and it's served me very well indeed.

> 1/2 head cauliflower

Simply put the cauliflower through your food processor using the shredding blade. This gives a texture that is remarkably similar to rice. You can steam this, microwave it, or even sauté it in butter. Whatever you do, though, don't overcook it! I usually put mine in a microwaveable casserole with a lid, add a couple of tablespoons of water, and microwave it for 7 minutes on high.

**YIELD:** This makes about 3 cups, or at least 3 to 4 servings. Assuming 3 servings, each with: 24 calories, trace fat, 2 g protein, 5 g carbohydrate, 2 g dietary fiber, 3 g usable carbs.


## Fauxtatoes

This is a wonderful substitute for mashed potatoes if you want something to put a fabulous sour cream gravy on! Feel free, by the way, to use frozen cauliflower instead. It works quite well here.

> 1 head cauliflower or 1 1/2 pounds (700 grams) frozen cauliflower
>
> 4 tablespoons (55 grams) butter

Steam or microwave the cauliflower until it's soft. Drain it thoroughly and put it through the blender or food processor until it's well pureed. Add the butter and salt and pepper to taste.

**YIELD:** 6 servings, each with: 72 calories, 8 g fat, trace protein, 1 g carbohydrate, trace dietary fiber, trace usable carbs. (This makes six generous servings.)

# The Ultimate Fauxtatoes

I'm not crazy about Ketatoes by themselves, but added to pureed cauliflower Fauxtatoes, they add a potato-y flavor and texture that is remarkably convincing! This is a killer side dish with many of your slow cooker main dishes.

1/2 head cauliflower
1/2 cup (50 grams) Ketatoes mix
1/2 cup (120 milliliters) boiling water
1 tablespoon (28 grams) butter

Trim the bottom of the stem of your cauliflower and whack the rest of the head into chunks. Put them in a microwaveable casserole dish with a lid. Add a couple of tablespoons of water, cover, and microwave on high for 8 to 9 minutes.

While that's happening, measure your Ketatoes mix and boiling water into a mixing bowl and whisk together.

When the microwave beeps, pull out your cauliflower—it should be tender. Drain it well and put it in either your food processor, with the S-blade in place, or in your blender. Either way, puree the cauliflower until it's smooth. Transfer the pureed cauliflower to the mixing bowl and stir the cauliflower and Ketatoes together well. Add the butter and stir till it melts. Add salt and pepper to taste and serve.

**YIELD:** 4 servings, each with: 140 calories, 5 g fat, 10 g protein, 14 g carbohydrate, 8 g dietary fiber, 6 g usable carbs.

# Index

# Acknowledgments

A few quick thank you's here:

To my darling friend Maria Vander Vloedt, who tested many, many recipes for this book. She's the perfect tester: She's smart and funny and reliable, she knows how to cook, she can follow instructions but make constructive suggestions when they're needed, she eats low-carb, and she has a husband and five kids to try my recipes out on! Thanks, Maria.

Also to my sister Kim, who is always up for a new recipe, and my pal Ray Stevens, who tested a bunch when crunch time rolled around: Thanks, guys!

As always, to my husband, Eric Schmitz. Thank God I married him, I could never find another person with his combination of skills in the open job market. All this, and he's nice to have around the house, too.

And to my editor, Holly, for browbeating me into writing this book. It's been a lot cooler than I expected.

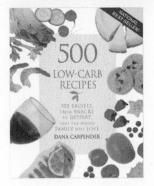

**500 Low-Carb Recipes**

ISBN 1-931412-06-5
$19.95/$28.95 CAN
Paperback, 500 pages
Available wherever books are sold

Okay, you've finally done it. You've gone low-carb! And no matter which one of the many low-carbohydrate diets you've chosen, you've discovered the joys of weight loss without hunger, not to mention energy that never seems to quit, and rapidly improving health.

**Just one little problem:** If you have to face one more day of eggs for breakfast, tuna salad for lunch, and a burger without the bun for dinner, you're going to scream. Worse, you're going to order a pizza!

Rejoice, my low-carb friend. Help is here; you hold it in your hands. In this book you'll find options galore. You'll find dozens upon dozens of new things to do with your protein foods and vegetables and you'll find recipes for foods you thought you'd never, ever be able to eat on your low-carb diet:

• Cinnamon Raisin Bread • Feta-Spinach Salmon Roast
• Sour Cream Coffee Cake • Obscenely Rich Shrimp
• Chocolate Mousse to DIE For • Mom's Chocolate Chip Cookies • Mockahlua Cheesecake
• French Toast • Heroin Wings • Sugar-Free Ketchup and Barbecue Sauce

You'll also learn more about how to count carbs and read labels, as well as get an overview of low-carb ingredients. You'll get the lowdown on all those new low-carb specialty products flooding the market. And, of course, you get 14 chapters of recipes, covering everything from Hors d'oeuvres, Snacks, and Party Nibbles, to Breads, Muffins, Cereals and Other Grainy Things.

You'll find cookies, cakes, and other sweets. Plus more recipes for main dishes and side dishes than you'll ever be able to eat your way through—everything from down-home cooking to ethnic fare; from quick-and-easy weeknight meals to knock-their-socks-off party food. So say goodbye to boredom, and hello to exciting low-carb meals every day! Whether you're a kitchen novice or a gourmet chef, you'll find dozens of recipes to suit your tastes, budget, and lifestyle.

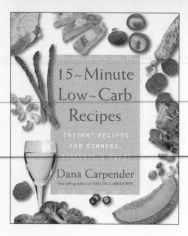

### 15-Minute Low-Carb Recipes

ISBN: 1-59233-041-X
$17.95/$24.95 CAN
Paperback; 256 pages

**Available wherever books are sold**

Yikes! It's 6:30 p.m., and you've just walked through the door after a long day at work, plus a couple of errands. You're tired, you're hungry—and before you can get your coat off, the family has started asking, "What's for dinner?"

In the past, you would have started boiling water for some quick mac-and-cheese, or warmed up a frozen pizza. Hungry and busy though you may be, you really don't want to trade your weight loss, high energy, and improved health for a quick-and-carb-y supper. What, oh what, to do?

Relax! No, really, sit down, relax, take a deep breath, and flip through *15-Minute Low-Carb Recipes*. You'll find dozens of wonderful family dishes that take no more than fifteen minutes to make, prep time included. You'll even find stuff you'd be happy to serve to company, should you be so brave as to invite people over on a weeknight!

So grab this book, and simplify your life. Instead of another round of plain steak or bunless fast food burgers, you could be eating:

Rosemary-Ginger Ribs with Apricot Glaze * Cranberry Burgers * Eggs Fu Yong
* Cumin Mushrooms * Swordfish Vera Cruz * Chicken Chili Verde
* Aladdin Salad * Beef and Bacon "Rice" with Pine Nuts
* Mexican Cabbage Soup * Aegean Chicken * Mushroom "Risotto"

And much, much more—all with the carbohydrate, fiber, and usable carb counts already calculated for you. What could be easier?

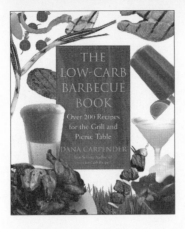

## The Low-Carb Barbecue Book

ISBN: 1-59233-055-X
$17.95/$24.95 CAN
Paperback; 256 pages

Available wherever books are sold

## BARBECUE!

Admit it, your mouth is watering at the very word. Who doesn't love a slab of succulent, smoky ribs, or moist, juicy chicken, hot off the grill and slathered in a sweet-and-tangy sauce?

Barbecue, with its generous helpings of protein, seems ideal for us low-carb types. But just take one glance at the ingredients of your favorite barbecue sauces and rubs—you might as well be pouring pancake syrup on your dinner! Then there are those traditional barbecue sides—potato salad, chips, sugary coleslaw, onion rings, and gallons of beer. Can't you feel your jeans getting tighter just thinking about it?

Well, help is at hand! In this book you'll find recipes for barbecue sauces that will turn your pork, chicken, or beef into pure ambrosia, and every single one of them contains half the carbs of traditional barbecue sauce, or less! You'll find sugarless rubs of every description, and mopping sauces to keep your meat moist and tender during that long, slow smoking.

Don't have time for traditional smoked barbecue? You'll find new, delicious, low-carb options for grilled meats, poultry, and fish, too. Plus, low-carb onion rings, hush puppies, salads, slaws, grilled veggies—everything you need to turn your barbecue into a low-carb summer feast. Even low-carb versions of your favorite summer cocktails!

### Recipes include:

Kansas City Barbecue Sauce * North Carolina Pulled Pork * Maple-Balsamic Glazed
Salmon * Five-Spice Beef Ribs * Chipotle-Garlic Grilled Asparagus
Bourbon-Molasses Barbecue Sauce * Apple-Maple Brined Ribs
Thai Grilled Chicken * Bodacious Brined and Barbecued Beef Brisket

So fire up the grill! It's time to barbecue!

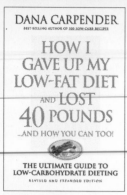

**How I Gave Up My Low-Fat Diet and Lost 40 Pounds**

ISBN 1-59233-040-1
$14.95/£9.99/$23.95 CAN
Paperback, 312 pages
Available wherever books are sold

It's time to go low-carb! Low-carbohydrate diets burn off twice the fat of low-fat or low-calorie diets, and they do it without making you starve. Here's the lowdown on how and why low-carbohydrate dieting works, not just for weight loss, but for dramatic health improvement. Without using boring, confusing medical jargon, I'll show you surprising research proving that carbohydrates, not fat, are the biggest culprit in causing diseases like diabetes, cancer, and coronary artery disease. Then I'll explain to you not one, but more than a half-a-dozen different approaches to cutting the carbs, and give you the information you need to mix-and-match these plans to come up with a low-carbohydrate diet you can live with for the rest of your long and healthy life.

So c'mon! Let me show you how to:

- Lose weight without hunger!
- Have the energy of a kid again!
- Eat more wonderful, real food than you ever thought possible!

All the while improving your cholesterol and triglycerides, lowering your blood pressure, and cutting your risk of diabetes and cancer. Let me tell you *How I Gave Up My Low-Fat Diet and Lost 40 Pounds . . . and How You Can Too!*

**Dana Carpender's Weight-Loss Tracker**

ISBN: 1-59233-151-3
$6.95/$9.95 CAN
Paperback; 128 pages
Available wherever books are sold

Struggling with your weight? Write down what you eat and watch the pounds disappear!

Most people think that meeting their weight loss goal begins and ends with what they put in their mouths. In reality, the majority of people who lose weight and keep it off have something else in common—they keep careful track of what they eat, especially carbs. *Dana Carpender's Weight-Loss Tracker* gives you all the information and space you need to write it all down: what you eat, how much, and each food's nutrient counts, including fiber, fat, protein, calories, and carbs. You can also record how much exercise you do and whether you're reaching your general health goals. Keeping track of this information will help you start your weight loss journey or bust out of a plateau!